HEALTHY
SUSTAINABLE
LIVING

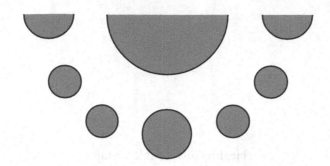

HEALTHY
SUSTAINABLE
LIVING

A Vision for the Future of Humanity

TOM BOUGSTY

iUniverse, Inc.
Bloomington

Healthy Sustainable Living
A Vision for the Future of Humanity

Copyright © 2012 Tom Bougsty

The information, ideas, and suggestions in this book are not intended as a substitute for professional advice.
Before following any suggestions contained in this book, you should consult your personal physician or mental
health professional. Neither the author nor the publisher shall be liable or responsible for any loss or damage
allegedly arising as a consequence of your use or application of any information or suggestions in this book.

iUniverse books may be ordered through booksellers or by contacting:

iUniverse
1663 Liberty Drive
Bloomington, IN 47403
www.iuniverse.com
1-800-Authors (1-800-288-4677)

Because of the dynamic nature of the Internet, any Web addresses or links contained in
this book may have changed since publication and may no longer be valid. The views
expressed in this work are solely those of the author and do not necessarily reflect the views
of the publisher, and the publisher hereby disclaims any responsibility for them.

Any people depicted in stock imagery provided by Thinkstock are models,
and such images are being used for illustrative purposes only.

Certain stock imagery © Thinkstock.

ISBN: 978-1-4759-6397-7 (sc)
ISBN: 978-1-4759-6398-4 (e)

Library of Congress Control Number: 2012922314

Printed in the United States of America

iUniverse rev. date: 11/30/2012

Contents

List of Figures

Acknowledgments

After graduation from Colorado State University with a Ph.D. in Psychology in 1980, my professional partner and spouse, Pru Marshall, and I opened a psychology and consultation practice in Cheyenne, Wyoming. We have one son, Skye Bougsty-Marshall.

I want to express my great appreciation to both Pru and Skye for their patience, support, and participation in relation to my decades of research, contemplation, and writing that has helped produce this book. In addition, I want to thank Marco Morelli for his competence with editorial and theoretical support and Jack Pugh for his cleansing of commas from the book. Staff members at iUniverse have been particularly helpful regarding editing and efficiency in the publication process. I owe special thanks to the many people I have seen as clients over the years who have helped me refine the quality and utility of the models, while the models served to help them understand and improve their lives.

Furthermore, I want to thank the authors listed in the reference section who work to cultivate conscious evolution and strive to create a better world. Finally, from an evolutionary perspective, I am grateful for the efforts of people throughout human history who have helped expand our consciousness and understanding of the world. Thanks to their efforts and to our entire evolutionary heritage, we now stand on the cutting edge of change in the world with the responsibilities to choose constructive evolutionary paths instead of destructive devolutionary ones as we cocreate the future.

Introduction

We face unprecedented challenges in the world today. The future of humanity will likely be determined by our responses to these complex issues. Unfortunately, our efforts to confront these challenges too often end in limited success. Consequently, people increasingly ask, "Are we heading in the wrong direction?" A more promising question to ask is this: "In what direction should we be heading?"

We can answer this latter question most comprehensively and productively by taking an evolutionary perspective. Approximately thirteen billion years ago, the Big Bang suddenly transformed the potential of all into manifest energy, information, and matter that began the processes of evolution. Metaphorically, as human beings we appeared on the scene in this "evolutionary movie" about 200,000 years ago. In these early years we faced an either/or choice to fit in or perish. Since we demonstrated extraordinary potentials for survival, creativity, and growth, we progressively acted in larger roles until we eventually emerged as the dominant player in the movie. As our innovative nature led to more success, we soon graduated from participating as mere players to acting increasingly like directors of the process. In this transition of our roles, the movie shifted from its inherent evolutionary script to appear more like a human script. We became the stars of the show. The story became about us and our survival, desires, and growth.

Therefore, we now act not only as players and increasingly as directors in the movie, but we have even advanced to take on the occasional role of producer. For instance, we have developed the capabilities to manipulate genes that have historically served as the evolutionary bridge for all life-forms to continue playing their unique roles in the world. In addition, we have garnered the ability to transfer millions of years of stored carbon from underground fossil fuels and release it into the atmosphere, thereby unintentionally modifying the climate of the planet. We have also learned to create technologies and introduce changes into the world to serve our special interests and short-term goals but have largely failed to notice the consequences of these changes for the other players, as well as for the evolutionary story itself.

If we intend to continue to survive and thrive, we must once again learn to fit into the larger processes of evolution upon which our life depends. We need to develop the skills to perceive from an evolutionary perspective, rather than simply from our personal and societal perspectives. Similarly, we need to develop the awareness, as well as the humility, to live in harmony with all that exists. This movie developed and evolved based on the participation and contributions of all the players—from subatomic particles to bacteria, from jellyfish to people. All the participants play important roles, although often unrecognized by humans, as they weave the web of life into a universal whole. Accordingly, we need to awaken to the reality that the movie belongs to all the players, and reciprocally, all the players belong to the movie. All serve important functions, or they would have already dropped out or been retired from the scene.

At this time, a profound leap from our normal human perspective to an evolutionary perspective is required. From this universal viewpoint, we can learn to play, direct, and produce for the benefit of all the players and the whole of reality. We can no longer afford our self-centered approach that primarily cares for our personal, group, and human needs. Our future depends upon the evolution of our consciousness, so we perceive, understand, and step into stewardship to protect and nurture the needs of all the players and the planet. In this way, we learn to respect and work in partnerships with all that share our journey and, ultimately, enable us to live. We realize that our best interests are inextricably grounded in the best interests of others, the planet, and evolution as a whole.

To meet this challenge, we need to develop a vision for the future that honors the ongoing flow of this remarkable evolutionary process, while also embracing the fundamental need for both the world and humanity to coexist. Since all the players have to function in a healthy manner to perform their roles proficiently, we need to conceptualize health comprehensively to include and promote the well-being of all. Furthermore, since evolution proceeds in creative, ever-changing ways that we only partially understand and predict, we need a precautionary approach to protect the players and their relationships from harm as we pursue an ultimate goal for sustainability.

I propose a vision for humanity in which we learn to live in harmony with the evolutionary movie. Five models introduce tools to help guide our efforts to play, direct, and produce in compatibility with this life-sustaining planetary process. These models depict universal features of humanity, thereby introducing opportunities to unite people throughout the world to work toward collective goals that simultaneously support our individual lives. Thus, the vision to create healthy sustainable living unites humans and planetary needs, so they operate coherently within the larger processes of evolution.

The first model provides a comprehensive overview of individual health. Since health provides the foundation for effective functioning, this model includes universal dimensions of human life that need to function, synergize, and balance to generate healthy living for the whole person.

The second model simply expands the first. It demonstrates that healthy living applies and needs to be developed across all levels of society, including families, businesses, communities, nations, and even the global community.

Third, an intervention model provides systematic choices about what combinations of these health dimensions, levels of society, and treatment, prevention, and wellness interventions generate healthy living.

Fourth, a universal ethical living model introduces how to evolve toward healthy living while protecting people and the planet from harm, such as from weapons of mass destruction and global pollution that can catapult us toward devolution instead of evolution.

Finally, a seven-step, healthy sustainable living model integrates the preceding models into a comprehensive approach to create our future. The whole process functions based on the underlying dynamics of the evolutionary impulse that creates ongoing changes in the universe through the processes of evolution, as portrayed in this integrative model. In the end, this model provides a methodology designed to work in increasing harmony with reality as a whole. Thereby, it helps us systematically guide our conscious evolution efforts toward a healthy sustainable future.

These models serve like maps on our evolutionary journey. They introduce screening tools to uncover the multiple sources that contribute to problems and then guide coordinated interventions to ameliorate the problems. In addition to improving problem solving, they provide tools necessary to help us grow and develop comprehensive healthy living. A healthy sustainable world depends upon healthy individuals, families, businesses, communities, and nations that all work together synergistically. To complement our efforts toward developing healthy living throughout the world, we also need to evolve our societal institutions such as our capitalist economy, our democracy, media, health care, and education systems to operate in service to the vision for healthy sustainable living.

The models provide progressively inclusive perspectives of reality that empower us to perceive and act in greater integrity with the world. In these ways, we cultivate sustainable living. This toolbox of models invites people worldwide to unite in service to the two fundamental motivations toward health and sustainability that lie at the heart of humanity and our future. Thus, we can mutually work to realize our highest human potentials, as we quest to cocreate our ultimate evolutionary destiny—healthy sustainable living for all.

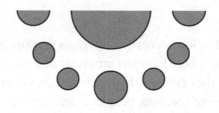

CHAPTER 1

Threats to the Future of Humanity

• • • • • • •

Solutions Depend upon Expansions in Our Consciousness

Numerous problems threaten our future, as indicated by the "Doomsday Clock" set at five minutes until midnight (Pappas and LiveScience, 2012). This clock portrays the precarious condition of humanity, as we live shockingly close to running out of time to solve the major problems that we face in the world. The clock shows that relative to a twenty-four hour day we have only five minutes left to learn to manage our problems. Environmental and financial crises, as well as political conflicts that can escalate into violence and wars, endanger our future. For instance, global climate change, ecosystem disruptions, and extinctions of plants and animals highlight environmental threats to our life-support systems. Meanwhile, modern culture depends upon financial systems that in 2007 shocked the world with a near-catastrophic meltdown. Such environmental and financial crises can stimulate or intensify political conflicts in which nuclear, chemical, biological, and cyber weapons exist and threaten us with mass destruction.

Ironically, while we have made remarkable progress in improving human life, we have inadvertently generated problems that now endanger our lives. This contradiction occurs largely due to our limited consciousness of reality. For example, we make progress in areas that we perceive as in our best interests (such as the generation and use of electricity based on fossil fuels resources). Beyond our immediate special interests, however, we sometimes unintentionally damage people and planetary systems that support our lives (for example, from the pollution and the depletion of fossil fuels).

Amazingly, we now stand as the greatest threat to our own future. Fortunately, we also stand as the greatest hope for our future. This hope arises from our capacities to expand our consciousness, so we perceive the world more accurately and fully, so we can choose actions that align with a sustainable future. At this time, we face probably the most important choice in human history. Do we continue our present approach to human progress that too often introduces threats to our continuing existence? Or do we choose to expand our consciousness so we learn to live responsibly in harmony with the world?

When we consider our various attempts to solve the problems we have created, we often see limited success. If we intend to develop successful solutions that protect and promote our future, we need to develop new approaches. Albert Einstein famously observed that we cannot solve problems by applying the same thinking that created them. Therefore, we must expand our consciousness so we understand reality and these complex problems with greater depth and breadth. Through increased comprehension, we can initiate effective actions to solve these intractable issues and, in the process, work more productively to create a healthy sustainable future.

Three Lenses through which We Perceive Reality

To live in harmony with the world, we must expand our consciousness, which requires understanding how to perceive reality more fully and accurately. We have three fundamental lenses, or perspectives, through which to perceive reality. These perspectives include:

1. The **lens of separateness** depicts reality as separate, material objects.

2. The **lens of relationships** reveals the interdependent exchanges of energy and information that occur beyond the surface appearance of these objects.

3. The **lens of oneness** unveils the separate objects and their relationships as components of a larger functioning whole.

We Perceive Reality Primarily through the Lens of Separateness

Through the lens of separateness we typically perceive material objects as the fundamental building blocks of reality. For instance, our sense organs detect specific frequencies of energy that our brain can convert into perceptions of separate, material objects. This process seems natural, since anything beyond the surface of our body appears separate from us. Thus, our evolutionary heritage and sense organs predispose us to perceive reality primarily through the lens of separateness in which distinct, material objects form the world. As a simple example, a fluffy cloud hangs in the blue sky above the apple tree that grows in the grassy field upon which we stand; our brain often perceives this reality as a collection of separate objects.

The other two perspectives provide information necessary to understand reality more fully and accurately. For instance, the second lens focuses on relationships. These relationships involve exchanges of energy and information that occur between, as well as serve to connect, material objects. Deepak Chopra said, "The physical world, the world of objects and matter, is made up of nothing but information contained in energy vibrating at different frequencies" (2003, 38). Thus, beyond the surface of material reality that we normally perceive, the world consists of interactive, interconnected relationships that involve energy and information exchanges.

Instead of existing simply as separate material objects, we also exist as energy and information in interdependent relationships. These relationships function at the core of our lives, yet they remain largely beyond our awareness when we focus through the lens of separateness. For instance in the previous cloud example, all the parts of the scene now exist connected in relationships. The cloud functions as part of the blue sky and can rain on the apple tree, the grass, and even on us, keeping us all alive. All exist in interconnected relationships that affect each other, despite also appearing as discreet separate objects.

A third perspective of reality reveals that material objects function in interconnected relationships that form larger wholes. From this lens of oneness, the whole contains the material objects and their interactive relationships in such a way that they form an interconnected oneness that is greater than the sum of its parts. The whole encompasses the parts and their relationships while organizing them into a more complex, orderly process.

Once formed, the whole can then serve as a part; it develops relationships with other parts of reality and can help form an increasingly larger whole. For instance, an atom consists of energy and information that can interact and combine with another atom to form a molecule. The molecule can eventually interact with other molecules to form a cell that functions as a whole greater than all its constituent molecules. Cells can then interact in relationships to form organs that interconnect to form organisms (Wilber, 1996). In the case of the cloud example, we now synthesize the separate objects and their relationships into a whole picture. Thus, we perceive the oneness of the entire scene, and in the process, detect reality more fully.

Throughout the universe, all the parts, including humans, function in relationships and participate in the whole evolutionary process. Ultimately, reality consists of the evolution of form that arises from the infinite, empty potential of universal intelligence. Many people describe this intelligent potential from which everything arises as God, or the Ground of Being according to some Eastern wisdom traditions (Wilber, 2006), or the zero point field (a ground-state energy field) in physics (McTaggart, 2002).

This infinite potential of the ground of being and the evolution of form in the universe prevail united as one—as the whole of "*reality*." Contained within this unified *reality* of all potential and all manifestation, we perceive a limited "personal reality" that detects only tiny portions of the overall *reality*. Nevertheless, we have the capacity to expand our personal reality to perceive progressively expansive versions of the oneness of *reality*. For instance, we can experience increasing versions of oneness when we connect and feel one with another person, and then expand our perspective to connect and feel one with a group of people. Similarly, we can expand our oneness experiences to connect with our community, nation, all humanity, with nature, and even with evolution. Ultimately, we have the capacity to awaken to our oneness with *reality* as a whole in which the infinite potential of the ground of being and the universe of manifest evolutionary form prevail in our awareness as nondual—unified as one whole.

As we experience more expansive versions of oneness, we perceive more of *reality*. In this process, we can integrate our separateness via our relationships to create and function in greater harmony with each of these larger wholes. As we perceive and act in cooperative oneness with our family, community, all humanity, and evolution, we tend to increase our coherence with *reality* overall.

The Perspective of Separateness Serves as an Incubator of Problems

Our predisposition to perceive *reality* in terms of separate objects provides only one perspective of what exists. This material perspective, however, has led to great achievements in the development of societies around the world. As Brian Swimme described, these developments have been so profound that human activity is now responsible for the majority of the evolutionary changes that occur on Earth (2010). For instance, our consciousness is estimated to double the information present each eighteen months (Wilson, 2009), and thereby, we rapidly change or evolve information and energy in the world. Meanwhile, our actions function like mutations that change the environment, especially apparent with material reality. Synthetic chemicals, innovative technologies, and urban development exemplify human creations that transform the world.

Yet, when we initiate actions from the lens of separateness, we can inadvertently damage the underlying relationships among the parts, as well as the functioning of the whole. From the perspective of separateness, our actions often appear appropriate; however, from the relationship and oneness perspectives our actions may be destructive. For example, when we act to serve the best interests of our self or our special interest group (as an expanded version of separateness), we can unknowingly and even sometimes intentionally harm or exploit others and the environment to meet our perceived needs. The eyes of separateness also predispose us to perceive differences, act competitively, and generate conflicts with other people, religions, nations, and even the natural environment (Global Oneness Summit, 2011). As a consequence, the separateness perspective contributes to or stimulates most of the problems we face in the world today (McTaggart, 2011).

When we interpret *reality* predominantly through only one of the three perspectives necessary for full, accurate perceptions, we can expect to create problems in our lives. Since the perspective of material separateness provides only a surface view of the world, we often change material reality without noticing the damages we inflict on the underlying relationships and their interconnections with the whole system. If we fail to value or even notice the relationship and oneness perspectives that are also essential for keeping us alive, we risk more than the major problems that we face today. If we continue to damage relationships among people and with other species and disrupt whole ecological systems upon which our lives depend, we unsuspectingly step into the role of perpetrators who may unknowingly bring about our own demise.

We Need to Integrate the Three Perspectives to Improve Our Perceptions of Reality

If we intend to survive and thrive in the future, we need to perceive *reality* as fully and accurately as possible and then act in harmony with the whole. Typically, this first requires expanding our consciousness so that our perceptions are more inclusive and complete. However, since the expansion of consciousness often requires considerable time and effort (Wilber, 2006), I will propose specific tools and methods to improve our efficiencies in perceiving and choosing actions that align with *reality*.

Along these lines, the models presented function like maps to guide us through territories that we fail to comprehend through normal awareness. They expand our state of consciousness so we perceive more of the world than usually available. For instance, the models will help us simultaneously perceive and integrate our separateness, interconnected relationships, and oneness with the whole. Such a comprehensive overview substantially improves our abilities to understand *reality* and minimize both intentional and unintentional harm in the world. We can then act to protect the life-support systems and the whole of *reality* upon which our future survival and success depend.

With this integrative approach, we can honor Einstein's wisdom to solve problems with expanded levels of thinking. As we increase our consciousness through the use of these models, we will significantly improve our perceptions and understanding of any issue of interest. When we better comprehend the complexities about how the world works relative to these three perspectives, we can initiate an evolutionary transformation in our ability to solve problems and create a sustainable future.

Without an increasingly full, accurate comprehension of *reality,* we may temporarily continue to make progress in meeting our separate special interests. Nevertheless, we will likely continue to undermine the relationships and the functioning of the whole that enables us to live. Eventually, such a special interest focus can stimulate enough unintended, destructive consequences to plunge us into a devolutionary cycle.

Consequently, as the primary leaders of evolutionary change on the planet, we face the challenge to either evolve or devolve. In devolution we can directly destroy humanity through wars and violence, for instance, or indirectly through pollution and disruptions of our life-support systems. To evolve we need to integrate the three perspectives of *reality* into a comprehensive approach that enables us to act in alignment with the evolutionary processes that make our lives possible. In other words, we need to learn to perceive and act as our separate self, who coexists in relationships with all people and the planet, and who cocreates for the benefit of all and the oneness inherent in *reality.*

Healthy Sustainable Living Models Guide Evolutionary Growth

The five, healthy sustainable living models incorporate these three perspectives as part of their core structure. This structural alignment with *reality* enables us to utilize the models to expand our consciousness, generate improvements in human functioning, and promote evolutionary growth.

The Healthy Living Model operates at the center of this new approach (see chapter 4). It introduces the foundation from which we can pursue the vision for healthy sustainable living to transform humanity to create a viable future. It provides the necessary tools for individuals to create healthy living in their personal lives that then serves as the springboard for healthy living on all levels of society.

The twelve universal dimensions of health that constitute the model need to all function, synergize, and balance to create healthy living. On the other hand, these dimensions also help us identify the different factors that contribute to the problems and unhealthy conditions in the world. We can then develop and coordinate comprehensive interventions that address the causes—and not merely the symptoms—of the problems. Furthermore, these dimensions reveal that cultural belief systems and societal institutions that traditionally account for our successes sometimes unknowingly contribute to the problems that threaten us. Along these lines, recommendations will be provided in this book about how to evolve our institutions such as our economy, democracy, media, health care, and education systems to support healthy sustainable living (see chapters 6 and 7).

To improve our efforts toward solving challenging problems, as well as continuing to promote healthy growth, the Societal Healthy Living Model emerges (see chapter 8). It takes the twelve dimensions of healthy living from the original model and applies them across all levels of society. In these ways, we can spread healthy living systematically throughout the global community as we improve healthy living on the individual, family, business, community, national, and world levels.

The societal model then expands into the Comprehensive Healthy Living Model. This provides a more in-depth means for identifying problems and what contributes to their existence. The contributions to problems often range across the twelve health dimensions and across all levels of society, from the personal to the community to the global levels. After identifying the major contributing factors to the problem, these contributors can be organized and prioritized. We can then select and design systematic actions across the three intervention modalities of treatment, prevention, and wellness (see chapter 8). In this way, we can expand, maintain, and restore health as appropriate to the situation. This comprehensive approach enables us to evaluate and intervene with the separate contributors, their interactive relationships, and the problem as a whole. Thereby, we incorporate all three perspectives of *reality* as we transform situations into healthier functioning.

The previous models function together to improve healthy living and at the same time cultivate and support sustainable living. Healthy living serves as a necessary foundation for sustainable living. Now we need a model to protect our evolutionary gains from possible destruction and devolution that could undermine healthy sustainable living. The Ethical Living Model introduces the methodology and the comprehensive overview of *reality* necessary to evaluate and then intentionally contribute to healthy living and sustainable living. This model extends healthy living across all levels of society to function in the context of five levels of evolution. This introduces an inclusive picture of *reality* as a whole (see chapter 9).

The Ethical Living Model provides the opportunity for us to evaluate whether our consciousness and actions contribute to evolution or devolution for humanity. This ability to analyze how much an action contributes to our lives or to our death provides a fundamental value system to guide our future conscious evolution. When an action appears to undermine our lives in the long-term, we have an ethical responsibility to protect the future of humanity. We avoid or stop or phase out any potentially devolutionary actions that may threaten the future of humanity.

Finally, an Integrated, Healthy Sustainable Living Model synthesizes these four previous models into a comprehensive approach to guide conscious evolution (see chapter 10). Through a seven-step process we systematically employ our highest consciousness to assess, evaluate, choose, and take actions that we then monitor. Thus, we have an ongoing planning process in which we promote healthy living, solve problems, and prevent devolutionary outcomes across all levels of the world. In this way, we can finally responsibly and ethically engage in conscious evolution.

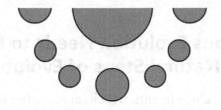

CHAPTER 2

The Processes of Evolution

Evolution Naturally Integrates the Three Perspectives of Reality

In traditional views, evolution proceeds through random mutations. Nevertheless, we now recognize that humans contribute to evolution through our consciousness and actions. Barbara Marx Hubbard calls this "conscious evolution" (1998). Successful evolution, based on changes in consciousness, depends upon the expansion of our awareness to perceive *reality* accurately enough so we can act increasingly in harmony with the natural processes of the universe.

We need to follow the general steps involved in evolution and model our actions on the successful processes that have brought the universe to this point. The particular evolutionary processes we need to follow convert separate forms through interconnected relationships to create progressively more complex wholes. Put another way, evolution integrates the "Separateness," "Relationship," and "Oneness" perspectives into a dynamic process of creation (see Figure 1).

Numerous authors (Hubbard, 2001; Dowd, 2007; McIntosh, 2007, 2012; Wilber, 2010; Hamilton, 2010; Elgin, 2010; Swimme and Tucker, 2011; Phipps, 2012; and Cohen, 2012) have noted directional tendencies in evolution. In general, "Evolution" progresses through a process of steps or phases portrayed in Figure 1. For instance, "Random Mutations" introduce "Creativity," which in turn produces "Competition" among the mutations as they participate in the natural selection processes. In general, the separateness perspective highlights these three phases of evolution. Thus, mutations, creativity, and competition frequently gain the most attention in discussions of evolution.

Nevertheless, "Cooperation" also represents an essential phase in the transformation of a mutation into a sustainable form. From the relationship perspective, the mutation must function cooperatively, in interaction with other forms, to contribute to the "Organization" necessary for evolutionary growth. The mutation then needs to stabilize into an ongoing "Order" in which it synchronizes to establish a more complex whole. In this way, the separate mutation operates in relationships to generate a complex, orderly whole, consistent with the "Oneness" perspective. Through such steps, evolution proceeds.

Conscious Evolution Needs to Mirror
the Natural Steps of Evolution

"Conscious Evolution" can introduce intentional changes, rather than merely random changes, into the processes of evolution. This major advance in evolutionary processes, in which humans lead the way, replaces random mutations (see the center of Figure 1) with "Consciousness" (see the center of Figure 2). Consciousness ultimately provides awareness of all *reality* through the unity of "Evolutionary Form + Empty Potential of All." In other words, we witness the oneness of all manifest form in evolution and the infinite potential of the ground of being and experience their unity in "Nondual Awareness" (Wilber, 2006). Such nondual awareness reveals our fundamental oneness with all and our most profound consciousness of *reality*.

Yet we typically perceive only very limited aspects of the whole of *reality*. We then convert our limited perceptions into a "Personal Reality." Our unique personal reality, synthesized from our particular time, place, and history of awareness, introduces "Creativity" into the world. Our unique consciousness generates "mutations" in information into the processes of evolution. We can then initiate "Personal Actions" in relation to our personal reality that can also affect evolution. Our actions can mutate not only information and energy, but also matter. The creativity generated by both our consciousness and actions quest for viability in the processes of natural selection. "Competition" among the new creations and existing separate forms, their relationships, and whole functioning systems then serve to help drive the selection processes. Accordingly, our ideas and behaviors contribute to the diversity important in selection processes to advance evolution toward greater complexity and order.

Again, "Cooperation" serves as a critical step in order for evolution to proceed. The new creation must participate in the complex relationships that already exist in the world. In this process, "Collective Cons(ciousness) & Actions" apply (see Figure 2). People share their consciousness to test the viabilities of the separate creation relative to different viewpoints and situational contexts. As a result, personal consciousness can expand into a collective consciousness from which others can take actions and participate in the creative process as well. In this phase of evolution the selection process progresses as cooperation serves as its primary driver.

The challenge then becomes how to integrate the creation into "Organization" with the existing environment. This requires multiple "Relationship Interconnections." If such relationships prove successful, then the creation needs to stabilize and maintain itself within the larger environment. This phase requires the development of "Relationship Interdependence," in which relevant evolutionary participants generate a more complex "Order" of mutual interactive functioning. When the creation finally evolves to serve as a part of a larger functional system, then the creation gains "Oneness" as a more complex whole. In this process, the initial personal creation transforms into an evolutionary creation.

In these ways, conscious evolution mirrors the basic processes of traditional physical and biological evolution (compare figures 1 and 2). In this case, conscious mutations, instead of random mutations, contribute to evolution. In other words, humans have the capabilities to alter evolution through our consciousness and actions and not depend merely on random changes.

Figure 1:
The Natural Processes of Evolution Integrate the Three Perspectives of Reality

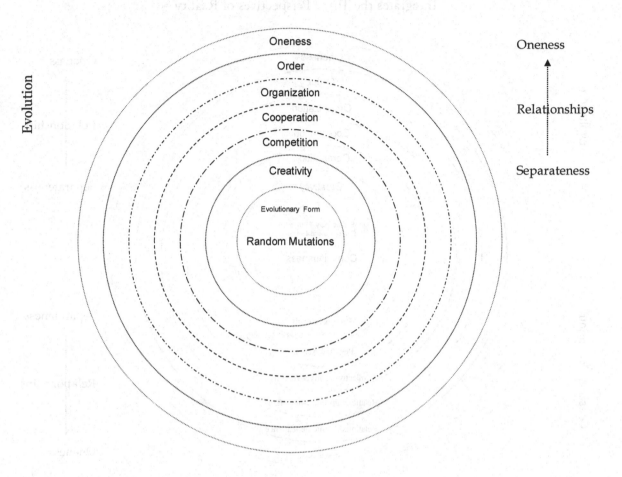

Figure 2:
Conscious Evolution Mirrors Evolutionary Processes and
Integrates the Three Perspectives of Reality

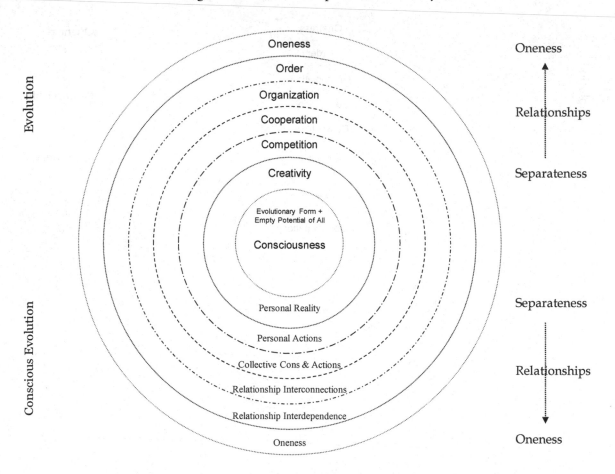

As an example, when our consciousness creates the belief (creativity) that we need the shelter of a new house, we can initiate actions to solicit competition among potential builders. The competition can lead to a cooperative relationship with a particular builder (collective consciousness and actions) who helps us organize (through relationship interconnections) and develop a collective sense of order that satisfies our wishes (relationship interdependence). The complexity of a new house then emerges from consciousness to be constructed into material reality. In these ways, we evolve from separateness through relationships with our consciousness and actions to create a more complex oneness. We construct a new house—random mutations have yet to accomplish this evolutionary feat.

Building a house, similar to creating any new material innovation, introduces potential risks regarding generating unintended devolutionary consequences. For instance, toxic spills or destruction of habitat for endangered species may occur in the house construction. Our power to cocreate, therefore, carries profound responsibilities for humans that must be embraced if we plan to develop a sustainable future. (These responsibilities will be discussed in more detail in chapters 9 and 10.)

Limited Awareness of Reality Can Shift Evolution into Devolution

Our awareness normally progresses from a self-centered, egocentric perspective of separateness to a group-centered, ethnocentric perspective (for instance, we expand our personal identity to our family, friends, community, or nation). Thus, we progress from a separateness lens into perceiving through a relationship lens. Although the ethnocentric perspective perceives more of *reality* than the egocentric view, extremely limited aspects of the whole are still detected.

When our consciousness expands to include the entire world, we shift into experiencing a "worldcentric" perspective. If we expand our consciousness further to include all *reality*, we extend into a "kosmocentric" perspective (Wilber, 2003). This all-inclusive lens has the capacity to perceive the evolutionary cosmos, as well as the ground of being. Thus, we have the potential to experience the unity of form and empty potential in a natural state of nondual oneness. We can perceive *reality* just as it is.

If we intend to live in harmony with *reality*, the kosmocentric perspective in which we perceive *reality* most fully represents our best hope for the future. Therefore, such pioneers in conscious evolution, including Andrew Cohen (2012), Craig Hamilton (2012a), Barbara Marx Hubbard (2011, 2012), Terry Patten (2012), Dan Brown (2006), Arjuna Ardagh, (2005), Candice O'Day (2012), Lola Jones (2009), and Peter Fenner (2009) teach methods to experience nondual consciousness. Although it is always available, nondual consciousness usually takes years of practice and meditation to awaken to, let alone stabilize as an ongoing experience in life.

Egocentric and Ethnocentric Perspectives Predispose an Unsustainable Future

Since the problems that we have created in the world demand immediate attention, we require additional creative methods to expand our consciousness. This need becomes especially crucial when we consider that nearly 70 percent of the world's population still perceives *reality* through the egocentric and ethnocentric viewpoints (Wilber, 2006) that invite an unsustainable future.

Egocentric and ethnocentric perspectives threaten our future sustainability in the following ways:

- Through egocentric and ethnocentric lenses we perceive too little of *reality* to choose how to live in harmony with the world.

- We perceive through the egocentric perspective what appears as "me versus the world;" meanwhile, we perceive through the ethnocentric perspective "us versus them" (Wilber, 2006). Hence, both views perceive relationships in terms of conflicts that naturally invite unsustainable consequences.

- We utilize self-interests and group-interests to guide our consciousness and actions. If we metaphorically portrayed *reality* as a puzzle, we naturally place our individual or group puzzle pieces in the center, as if all the other pieces should serve us as we operate at the center of the world.

- Special interests that inherently exist in egocentric and ethnocentric perspectives require competition with others and the world. We need to compete, and if necessary or convenient, exploit other parts of the puzzle for our interests.

- Since evolution proceeds based on competition shifting into cooperation, the egocentric and ethnocentric perspectives trap us in our self and our group. We tend to compete with everything beyond our special interests which undermines the cooperation necessary to evolve the world toward a sustainable future.

- We assume that others perceive the world the same as us, so if everyone would just take responsibility for themselves then all would be fine. Unfortunately, if we all used only special interests to guide our behaviors, collective interests of humanity and the planet would be ignored and likely be further exploited.

- We fail to perceive beyond our self- and group-interests from the egocentric and ethnocentric perspectives. Therefore, we fail to notice the damages and harm that we inadvertently or intentionally inflict on others and the planet in pursuit of our personal and group concerns.

- Without recognizing the damages that we inflict upon our life-support systems, we fail to take responsibility for our consciousness and actions and, thereby, fail to grow into healthy sustainable living.

- We fail to perceive from the worldcentric perspective in which we exist in a web of interdependent relationships and global oneness. Self-interests in this context mean that we care for ourselves by also caring for all people and the whole world.

Worldcentric and Kosmocentric Perspectives Are Essential for Sustainability

The worldcentric level of consciousness represents the minimal level of awareness necessary to create a sustainable future (Wilber, 2006). Fortunately, the models introduced beginning in chapter 3 provide a temporary means to awaken to a worldcentric—and even a Kosmocentric—perspective. As a result, people throughout the world have the opportunity to expand their consciousness to help create a sustainable future.

Until we develop worldcentric and kosmocentric perspectives, we will continue to initiate creativity and actions from the egocentric and ethnocentric perspectives. Since these two viewpoints focus on our self and our group (whether family, ethnic, corporate, or nation), they perceive the world predominately through the separateness perspective and partially through the relationship perspective. From the vantage-point of evolution portrayed in Figure 3, they generate "Special interest Creativity" and "Special interest Actions." Since special interests mean that we prioritize individual and group interests over the concerns of humanity, the world, and *reality*, we naturally ignore and sometimes exploit whatever exists beyond our area of concern. "Conflicts with *Reality*" then frequently arise, as we perceive only small portions of the relationship and oneness realms.

Special Interests Threaten the World with Devolution

We can perceive some of these conflicts on the world scene when we notice the feedback provided by protesting, impoverished, and suffering people around the world. Similarly, we can perceive the damages done to the air, water, and land environments of the planet. As a result of such conflicts, "Relationship disruptions" increasingly threaten the world with "Disorganization," "Disorder," and "Destruction." Ultimately, wars, pandemics, and global changes in biodiversity and ecosystems heighten the potential for "Chaos" and death in the future.

When we act based on our egocentric and ethnocentric separate interests, evolution may appear to advance. Yet beneath the surface, the relationships and the oneness of the whole that enables these separate interests to exist can suffer damages. As a result, evolution proceeds on the surface, while "Devolution" undermines our progress under the surface. This means that our limited perceptions of *reality* can generate special interest creativity that serves our immediate desires, but may ultimately initiate processes that lead to chaos and destruction.

An example of this devolutionary process involves the development of new technologies used in commercial fishing. These advanced, special interest methods catch so many fish that over-fishing can result. Other species are often killed and ecological damages accumulate to the ocean environment and ecosystems upon which the remaining fish depend. The devolution of fish species and populations along with their natural environments now threaten many fishing operations and their ability to continue feeding people around the world.

What appears through the separateness lens as evolution on the surface of the material world can generate devolutionary processes in the relationship and oneness lens of *reality*. Whenever we operate from special interest concerns perceived through the separateness lens, we commonly fail to consider the long-term ramifications for all people and the planet. This means that most technologies pass the cultural evolution test in which the technology immediately meets a perceived need in the society. Nevertheless, we often neglect to consider the various relationships beyond our specific concern that can lead to long-term, destructive consequences for humanity and the planet. As a result, many modern innovations place us at different degrees of risk for devolution. For instance, fossil fuels as our primary energy source that underlies most technologies as well as the development of modern society will be examined in chapter 9 to provide an overview of its numerous evolutionary and devolutionary consequences.

Figure 3:
Evolutionary Processes Can Shift into Devolutionary Processes
Due to Our Limited Awareness of Reality

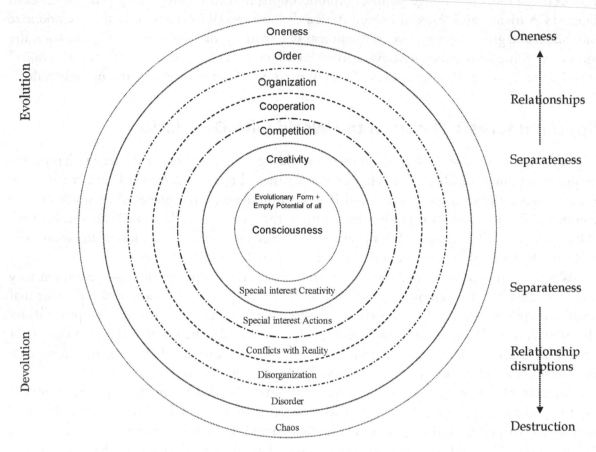

A Practical Example—Evolutionary versus Devolutionary Reactions in This Book

Consistent with the different phases of evolution we can develop a simple screening tool to evaluate if we respond to a situation in an evolutionary or devolutionary way. The phases of evolution portrayed in Figure 2 include consciousness stimulating creativity, competition, cooperation, organization, order, and oneness. These phases convert separateness experienced primarily through the creativity and competition phases into relationships that occur in the cooperation, organization, and order phases. Interdependent relationships of separate objects can then integrate into oneness that forms a more evolved whole. Sustainable evolution depends upon reaching this oneness phase that provides a stable platform from which further evolution can proceed.

In conscious evolution, we face the challenge to shift beyond our normal perceptions of separateness. We need to expand our awareness from the competition into the cooperation phase to participate consciously with the relationships that support our lives. In other words, the transition from competition into cooperation represents a critical bridge to cross if we intend to activate positive conscious evolution.

As a practical example, we can explore how to apply this evolutionary process in the reading of this book. For instance, my foremost intention in writing the book is to contribute to conscious evolution that shifts us toward healthy sustainable living. With this goal in mind, I have developed my personal reality relative to many aspects of the collective reality of others, as well as from glimpses into other aspects of *reality*. The action to publish this book and share my current limited views of *reality* represents an effort to introduce some creative mutations into what already exists. Naturally, this information will compete with other views.

Thus, I have attempted to organize and unify what appears as several universal components within *reality* and present these materials in manners that optimistically invite cooperation. My hope is that the competition phase will prove more productive and efficient, if we intentionally evolve our perspective into the cooperative phase first. This means we choose to have respectful, caring exchanges in relation to our differences; we listen and learn from each other rather than compete in win-lose exchanges.

We choose to operate based on a win-win approach to our relationship. In the process, we can discuss, understand, and organize our differences in efforts to develop more accurate and effective perceptions of *reality*. We can then more easily and productively organize our mutual creativity into increasing order. Eventually, we may unify our consciousness into a shared reality in which we act as one, or at least act for achieving a greater oneness. In this way, we can then cocreate using collective efforts to contribute to conscious evolution that moves us toward healthy sustainable living.

Nevertheless, the limitations inherent in my personal reality, creativity, as well as my limited abilities to express these can invite competition. Such reactions can involve who is right and wrong or who will win and lose based on our different perceptions. This natural competition occurs when we perceive something different than what we believe—or worse, we perceive something as incorrect relative to our personal reality, especially if it appears to be a threat to our identity or safety.

If you happen to find that you react in competitive, resistive manners to the different conceptualizations I present in this book, consider this normal reactivity. On the other hand, if you find yourself responding with openness and a cooperative sense of wanting to learn and share commonalities and differences to better understand and further develop the concepts, then you have shifted into a higher evolutionary process.

Your natural egocentric and ethnocentric perspectives have, at least temporarily, been largely transcended. Your response may originate from a worldcentric or kosmocentric perspective in which improved approximations of the truth occur. From such perspectives we progressively move beyond the viewpoints that "I am right" or "my group's collective belief system is right."

Walking the Evolutionary Path

In this light, I propose this method as a simple tool to evaluate our evolutionary path-walking. In any situation, we can simply notice if we respond through competition or cooperation. If we react with competition and resistance, we likely perceive through an egocentric or ethnocentric lens. These special interest perspectives attempt to serve our particular personal or group levels of concern. Nevertheless, since these viewpoints omit most of *reality*, while their impacts ripple throughout the world, the results will in the end likely stimulate devolutionary outcomes.

In other words, when we compete for our personal and group interests, we may win on the surface while the competition loses. Yet when the competition loses, the relationship and the oneness functions will naturally lose to some extent. When enough losses occur in a relationship and in the functioning of the whole, destruction increasingly results. Consequently, the separate winners, who also live interdependently within the relationships and the whole, are unsuspectingly harming themselves.

In contrast, if we perceive consistent with the intention of cooperation, we open the door to access *reality* more fully and participate with it and other people as partners. We respect that unique creativity functions as a necessary step in evolution. We welcome the exploration of differences and unique creations in efforts to organize higher orders of creativity through cooperative, growing relationships. In the process, we enhance our opportunities to realize greater oneness on the evolutionary path.

Thus, we step into the role of cocreators. In addition, we model and encourage the evolution of collective consciousness with others. Through such cooperation, instead of striving to win over the competition, we shift from our normal eyes of separateness into our eyes of relationships and oneness. In the process, we engage in conscious evolution that moves us toward a healthy sustainable future for humanity.

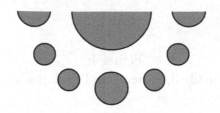

CHAPTER 3

Five Models for Healthy Sustainable Living

• • • • • • •

The Models Expand Consciousness so We Act in Increasing Harmony with Reality

We need to prioritize the development of our consciousness into the worldcentric and kosmocentric perspectives in order to live in integrity with *reality*. When we lack consistent access to these expanded perspectives, we need perceptual tools to help us operate at these levels so we can consciously avoid devolution.

I propose three core models, accompanied by a supplemental intervention model and an integrated summary model. Each model supports our continued evolution while providing increasingly inclusive perspectives of *reality*. Along these lines, the models temporarily expand our consciousness. They also portray the combination of our separate, relationship, and oneness natures. This comprehensive template helps us perceive *reality* more accurately and fully, so we can perceive and act to avoid devolution as we continue on our evolutionary journey.

Each model includes separate dimensions of health that interact in complex relationships that ultimately form progressively larger wholes. The oneness nature of the whole integrates these separate health components and their interactive relationships; it forms increasingly complex orders of healthy living. As a result, each model facilitates our conscious evolution to perceive and act in manners that develop increasingly comprehensive health.

In the initial model we evolve as individuals into healthy living. The second model promotes healthy living across all levels of human society, while the third model enables us to choose wellness, prevention, and remediation interventions to improve health systematically throughout society. The fourth evolutionary model shows how healthy living depends upon the health of all people, the planet, and all levels of evolution. See Figure 4 for a pictorial overview and outline of how models 1 ("Individual Health"), 2 ("Societal Health"), and 4 ("Evolutionary Health") interface that will be described in greater detail in later chapters.

Figure 4:
Integration of Individual, Societal, and Evolutionary Health Models

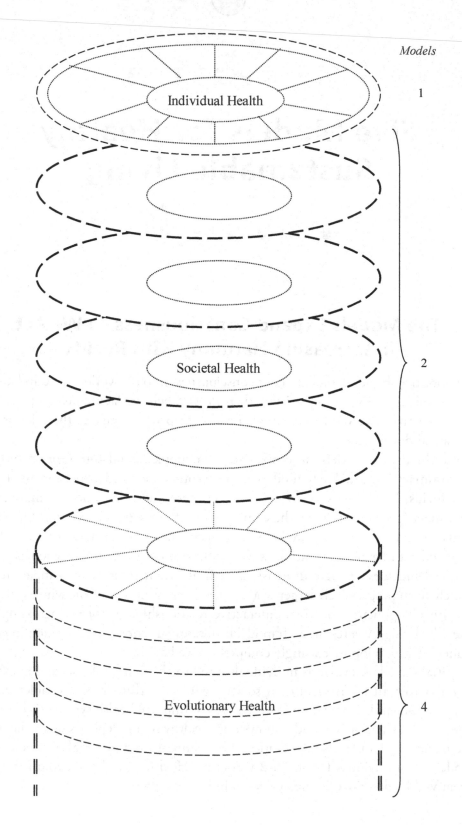

In combination, the models demonstrate the need to pursue healthy living and simultaneously integrate health across the individual, human, and evolutionary levels. Since the models nest together with the first contained within the second, and the initial two contained within the fourth model, each affects and depends upon the others. The first model focuses on individual health that includes the twelve dimensions of healthy living that support the same dimensions throughout all levels of the global community in the second, societal health model. Reciprocally, healthy living on all the societal levels (family, business, community, nation, and global) need to support individual health.

In a similar fashion, the first two models that involve the individual and all levels of humanity need to function productively to promote health in the evolutionary model that expands to include the planet and evolution. Important to note is that individual health sits atop societal health, which functions dependent on evolutionary health. Although all function interdependently, individual health exists only when societal health and evolutionary health support it. This means that we function at the top of the evolutionary world, and therefore, we stand at greater risk of devolution. No significant destruction can occur to society or evolution without threatening our existence.

Therefore, we have to learn to function as healthy individuals, but we simultaneously have to contribute to health throughout all levels of society and all levels of evolution. In other words, if we shift from our normal separateness perspective into relationship and oneness perspectives, we expand our view of our individual self into a social self and an evolutionary self. In the fullness of our existence we then recognize the need to work on behalf of our whole self in which we benefit our separate, interconnected, and interdependent oneness.

Successful conscious evolution also depends on the integration of the separate, relationships, and oneness perspectives. This integration of these perspectives needs to occur internally within each model and externally linking all the models. Each model integrates these evolutionary perspectives within its structure, as seen more clearly in the later presentations of each specific model (as separate health dimensions interact in relationships to form healthy living as a whole).

Meanwhile, external integration occurs when we combine the initial individual model (representing separateness) with the second societal model (depicting relationships) in the context of the universal fourth model (of the oneness of the world and *reality*). These models reflect natural evolutionary processes that provide internal evolution within each model and external evolution among the models as they interface with the world. Cooperative processes within and between the models that operate congruent with evolutionary processes support our capabilities for developing a healthy sustainable future.

Our Brain Fails to Perceive All the Important Components of Our Lives

Each model portrays separate aspects of human life that interrelate to develop our personal and collective capabilities. Although a relatively simple depiction, each model facilitates perceptions of how the separate parts of our lives interact to create a healthy person, business, or society. The interdependent relationships involved often function beyond our awareness. Concurrently, we similarly fail to notice most of the separate components as we typically focus on only one or two. This occurs largely because our brain consciously perceives only about four to six items at one time (Hanson, 2012). In other words, we simply lack the natural capacity to perceive simultaneously all the important areas that contribute to our lives.

Consequently, we need a method to compensate for this fundamental limitation of our brain. The method employed here identifies those separate items critical for healthy functioning then organizes these items into categories of increasing complexity. Our brain can then perceive the larger categories, while also accessing the individual items contained within each category. In this way, the models include the major separate parts and their interconnected relationships that contribute to a transcendent whole. This transcend-and-include approach (Wilber, 2006) enables us to expand our consciousness, at least temporarily, so we can perceive separateness, relationships, and the whole in one pictorial form.

Metaphorically, these models appear similar to puzzles. Separate puzzle pieces depict different aspects of the world that fit together and dynamically interact. The combination of separate pieces and their interconnected relationships generate increasingly comprehensive configurations of *reality*. In addition, the first model then becomes a piece in a larger, more inclusive second model that, in turn, assimilates into the fourth, universal model. In this way, we can analyze how an action taken in one area can affect other pieces of the puzzle, as well as affect the other interconnected puzzles. Thus, this methodology enables us to integrate the separate, relationship, and oneness perspectives, so we can choose responsible actions that function in greater integrity with evolutionary processes and all aspects of *reality*.

The Models Depict Universal Features of Humanity

To maximize our capacity to perceive *reality* accurately, the models include the major dimensions of life that contribute to our healthy functioning. Partial perceptions of our life provide only partial answers and, more importantly, leave us unaware of damages that we may initiate that undermine our life-support systems.

To optimize the utility of the models, these universal dimensions of health operate across universal levels of the global community. In this capacity, the models expand from applying to the individual to apply to all collective levels of society that range from the local to the community to the global levels. As a result of the universal nature of the health dimensions as well as the universal levels of society, people throughout the world have a common ground upon which to cooperate to achieve goals for healthy living. In this process, they can value and benefit separate individuals, collective groups, all humanity, the planet, and the whole of *reality*. In addition, the models and methodology create opportunities to develop comprehensive visions to guide us toward achieving our highest potentials so we can create a viable future.

The Universal Motivation for Sustainable Living

All people want to survive under normal circumstances. Similar to other living organisms, sustainable living represents a natural, universal drive. For instance, our evolutionary brain contains an organ called the amygdala, which defaults our awareness to save our life with fight, flight, or freeze reactions whenever we perceive ourselves to be in danger (MacLean, 1990). This brain default automatically operates to save our life and prevents us from choosing death, except in extreme cases of suffering. In addition to this brain predisposition that functions to protect our survival in mortal life, we seem predisposed to quest for sustainability in relation to eternal existence.

Throughout human history, religious traditions have developed to help explain eternal life or offer it as an outcome for obeying specified moral codes. Fortunately, we have the potential to learn to access our eternal nature whenever we witness and experience our oneness with the infinite potential of the ground of being (Cohen and Wilber, 2004; Cohen, 2012). Ultimately, this universal drive for sustainable living guides us as individuals and as a species to survive and perpetuate life. Consequently, a vision for the future of humanity needs to place this universal motivation for sustainability at its core.

The Universal Motivation for Health

The second universal motivation of humanity incorporated into all the models involves healthy living. All people value their health as they attempt to grow, maintain, and enjoy their lives. Health serves as a natural motivator, especially when considered in relation to its alternative—sickness. Moreover, health represents a necessary component for sustainable living as it minimizes pain, suffering, and ultimately death. Overall, our health serves three major purposes in evolution:

1. to avoid pain, destruction, and death;

2. to maintain, stabilize, and preserve life; and

3. to promote happiness and personal, societal, and evolutionary growth.

Healthy Sustainable Living Provides a Guiding Vision for the Future of Humanity

A vision for the future of humanity requires at least the following features. The vision must:

- Embrace all of *reality*, including the perspectives of separateness, relationships, and oneness as we participate as part of the nondual whole;

- Help us evolve in harmony with the natural processes of evolution (consciousness, creativity, competition, cooperation, organization, order, and oneness);

- Apply universally to people throughout the world;

- Enliven universal motivations for health and sustainability to empower people to act in integrity with *reality*; and

- Introduce ethical guidelines to manage our conscious evolution efforts, so we promote growth and avoid devolutionary outcomes.

The vision for healthy sustainable living, accompanied by its models, integrates these crucial features. For instance, healthy living for individuals and society in the context of evolution requires us to perceive and act increasingly in harmony with *reality*. In the process, healthy living supports sustainable living, as we bridge all past generations with future generations so our progeny can continue on this remarkable evolutionary journey. The universal motivations for health and sustainability create the potential to unite people throughout the world to work for mutual, higher purposes. When guided by assessment and intervention information that emerges from these models, people can become motivated to participate constructively in conscious evolution. The vision creates the opportunity and provides guidance on how to engage in conscious evolution that prevents harm and devolution, as we serve the higher purpose to create a viable future for humanity and the world.

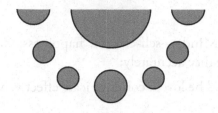

CHAPTER 4

The Healthy Living Model

• • • • • • •

Introduces a Foundation for Healthy Sustainable Living

Healthy living needs to include all the major dimensions of life that contribute to health. Traditionally, health has been conceptualized narrowly, consistent with the perspective of separateness and with our limited conscious capacities to perceive only four to six items at once. Because of this, we have failed to appreciate the multiple factors involved in health, as well as their synergistic relationships that generate health as a whole. For instance, the physical health of a person has been a traditional focus. Meanwhile, in the last fifty years, mental health has received increasing attention, although still significantly underappreciated. More recently, economic crises have stimulated greater interest in economic health. Nonetheless, health as a whole needs to include all the major dimensions of life which contribute to developing a healthy person.

In this book, health involves twelve dimensions of life that work together to generate overall health. These twelve separate areas of human life interact to form the Healthy Living Model (see Figure 5; also see Bougsty, 2012 for how to develop a personal plan and lifestyle to create healthy living). In general, each dimension must contribute to the growth and maintenance of our lives. These components operate in interdependent relationships to support healthy living. Thus, healthy functioning in each area works in concert with a dynamic balance among the different dimensions, so the separate components and their relationships integrate to form a whole healthy person. If one or more of the dimensions experience neglect or perform in dysfunctional manners, negative effects can spread through the interconnected, interdependent relationships. Other dimensions, as well as the overall health of the person, can suffer.

Twelve Major Health Dimensions Contribute to Human Health

The Healthy Living Model consists of the following twelve health dimensions:

- Physical health (Body)—healthy eating, exercise, relaxation, sleep, sex, safety, and health care;

- Psychological health (Mind)—self-esteem; happiness; mind management of brain functions to perceive reality accurately;

- Family health—love and be loved; communicate effectively; create a sense of "family;" model healthy living;

- Social health—social esteem, close friends; communicate with empathy, honesty, and nonviolently in win-win relationships; create/use healthy social institutions;

- Cultural health—appreciate human creations such as art, music, cultural norms, laws, and worldviews;

- Vocational health (Work)—productive, satisfying work/school/chores;

- Economic health (Money)—earn a living and balance savings, consumption, and contributions;

- Political health (Power)—set goals, make healthy choices, influence others, and manage the twelve dimensions of health;

- Recreational health (Play)—personal interests, hobbies, humor, and enjoyable activities;

- Environmental health—safe/comfortable home, community, world; minimize harm; and appreciate natural settings and public services;

- Spiritual health—connect with a "higher power;" experience purposes and gratitude in life; meditate, awaken to our oneness with all; and

- Ethical health—seek and tell the truth as we perceive it; contribute to others, the planet, and the oneness of all, so healthy living continues.

Each Health Dimension Needs to Function in Healthy, Balanced Manners

Each of these dimensions needs to function in healthy manners, interact in complementary relationships, and balance as an orderly whole to optimize health. In other words, personal health depends upon an integration of the three perspectives of *reality* (separateness, interconnected relationships, and overall oneness). When we utilize this model, we can operate in greater integrity with *reality*. For instance, the model naturally expands our consciousness, as we perceive twelve major dimensions that contribute to our health. Normally, our brain limits our conscious awareness so we cannot perceive nearly this many separate items at one time. Furthermore, the model portrays that these separate dimensions function in interdependent relationships that exchange energy and information beyond our usual awareness. Finally, we can perceive our health as a whole that encompasses each of the separate dimensions and their interconnected relationships. Thus, our overall health known as healthy living constitutes more than the sum of its parts, similar to all evolutionary wholes.

Figure 5:
The Healthy Living Model

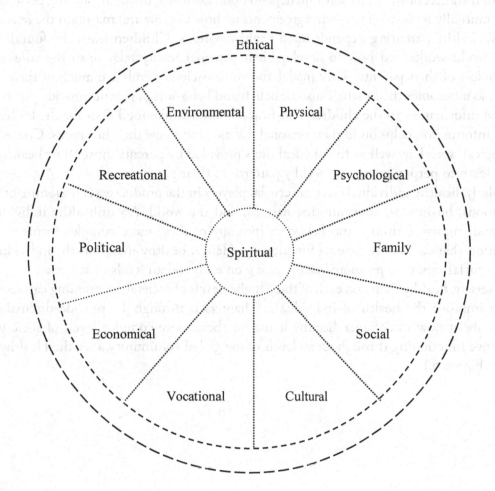

Individual and Societal Healthy Living Work Reciprocally

Healthy living in individuals lays the foundation for healthy living throughout society and the world. For instance, healthy relationships depend upon healthy individuals sharing personally and working mutually to develop win-win agreements on how to grow and maintain the relationship. Similarly, healthy parenting depends upon healthy parents. Children learn the foundations of how the world works and how to develop their personal reality relative to the consciousness and behaviors of their parents. They model and subconsciously embrace much of their parents' behavior, so it becomes their own. Thus, the beliefs and behaviors of parents provide psychological and social information to the children that function almost like food does for the body; in this case, the information helps build their personal realities and shape their behaviors. Consequently, psychological, social, as well as the physical diets provided by parents must all be healthy or the children learn to perpetuate the unhealthy patterns of their parents.

Similarly, healthy individuals serve as crucial players in the productive functioning of healthy organizations, businesses, communities, nations, and the world. An unhealthy individual can introduce disruptive attitudes and behaviors into any of these more complex forms of human organization that can undermine its functioning. Hence, healthy living on the individual level provides crucial inputs to promote healthy living on each and all levels of society.

Conversely, healthy living on each of these higher levels of societal functioning can reciprocate and help improve the health of individuals. Chapters 6 through 10 provide discussions and examples about how to enhance healthy living on these more complex levels of society, so we can improve functioning throughout all levels of the global community. (See the Healthy Living Model in Figure 5.)

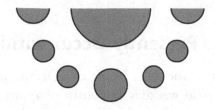

CHAPTER 5

Unhealthy, Unsustainable Conditions Exist in Our Present Society

• • • • • • • •

Cultural Beliefs and Practices Sometimes Limit Our Health

We can examine the "American Dream" for prosperity and success as an example of an important cultural belief that has generated great achievements and, sometimes inadvertently, undermined our health and sustainability. The American Dream has served to motivate and activate citizens to achieve tremendous accomplishments in the development of the nation, as well as indirectly in the world. However, these outstanding successes in technological and cultural development have sometimes been accompanied by unintended collateral damages, such as those described later in this chapter. As a result, the American Dream has traditionally been noted for its great successes, while recently it has received increasing attention for problems it sometimes generates.

To better understand how unintentional destructive consequences could accompany this successful cultural belief, we can simply examine the American Dream of success in relation to the healthy living model. From the perspective of the twelve dimensions of healthy living, this amazingly productive dream reveals its pathways to success, as well as uncovers a number of inherent limitations. For instance, the American Dream typically prioritizes the "vocational (work)," "economic (money)," and "political (power)" dimensions in efforts to achieve success. In other words, if we work hard, we will earn the money and gain the power to buy whatever we want. In this process, we achieve success. The dream ideally culminates with retirement from the work dimension as we shift into the "recreational (play)" dimension.

The major problem regarding success in this conceptualization of *reality* is that only three (work, money, and power) of the twelve health dimensions are prioritized. This leaves the other nine dimensions as secondary and sometimes vulnerable to neglect or exploitation. The apparent assumption is that success with work, money, and power will lead to success throughout life. Yet success in each area depends on having enough time and energy to develop the necessary awareness and skills to perform effectively in each area. Without adequate investment of time and energy in three-fourths of the health dimensions, they naturally struggle to maintain their viability and avoid destructive outcomes. As a consequence, overall health frequently suffers.

Unhealthy Problems Presently Occur within Each Dimension

We can examine the demands that the three "American Dream dimensions" make on our time and energy. If we imagine a typical weekday to consist of approximately eight to ten hours at work plus commuting, eight hours for sleep, three hours for eating, personal care, and household chores, as well as three hours for shopping and television watching, only zero to two hours remain to invest in the other nine dimensions. When we invest so minimally in such important areas of our life as our body, mind, family, environment, and spiritual health, problems for healthy living naturally develop.

For instance, each dimension of health currently suffers from significant problems in the United States, such as the following examples show:

- Physical health—more than two-thirds of the population is overweight (Centers for Disease Control and Prevention—CDC, 2008);

- Psychological health—stress affects nearly everyone and secondarily contributes to various chronic diseases (ScienceDaily, 2007);

- Family health—half of marriages end in divorce (CDC, 2009a);

- Social health—one in one hundred Americans are imprisoned; the United States has almost one-quarter of all the world's prisoners despite having only 5 percent of the world's population (Liptak, 2008);

- Cultural health—an emphasis on individual rights and independence often favors and protects personal and special interests at the expense of relationships, the public, the planet, and the whole of *reality*;

- Vocational health—nearly 9 percent of the adult population has been unemployed during the great recession (Bureau of Labor Statistics, 2011), while the total underutilized labor force has been approximately 15 percent (Bureau of Labor Statistics, 2012);

- Economic health—the top 1 percent control 42 percent of the wealth in the United States (My Budget 360, 2011); 22 percent of children younger than eighteen lived in poverty in 2010 (US Census Bureau, 2010);

- Political health—a plutocracy, in which the wealthy rule, has largely replaced our democracy (Hartmann, 2004; see later discussions in chapter 7 on how to improve our democracy);

- Recreational health—violence, sex, and sports encourage materialistic entertainment over informational, relationship, and whole-systems entertainment;

- Environmental health—global changes disrupt the climate, oceans, water supplies, gene pools, and the survival of species;

- Spiritual health—only one hour per week is often allocated to spiritual practices;

- Ethical health—greed and inequality contributes to "the haves and have-nots," as well as to the financial crises, wars, and a country and world dominated by money.

The American Dream Undermines Itself by Neglecting Healthy Sustainable Living

The traditional goal of the American Dream for success effectively promotes economic development and special interests. Yet in the process, it can harm the universal and personal goals for healthy sustainable living. These unintended consequences can be predicted when we view the situation from the perspective of healthy living. For instance, when we prioritize separate parts (such as work, money, and power) over the whole (all twelve dimensions), dysfunctions naturally result. Anytime separate, special interests take precedence over the whole, neglect and risks of harm and exploitation occur to the whole. Ironically, the success achieved in the American Dream dimensions is often undermined by problems that develop in the other nine dimensions.

A deficiency in any dimension can contribute to problems in other areas, since these dimensions operate in interdependent relationships. Therefore, problems in our personal, social, environmental, spiritual, and ethical areas of life can undermine functioning in the American Dream dimensions. We commonly see that physical and mental health problems, as well as family and social conflicts, interfere with productivity at work. Environmental problems can also interfere with workplace productivity while ethical problems can help plunge the financial system into a great recession. When we focus so intensely on the dream dimensions of work, money, and power, we neglect the health of many other dimensions. As these other dimensions suffer, they can impair the productivity and success of the American Dream.

Neglect of Other Health Dimensions Result in Enormous Economic Costs

While the economic costs of dysfunctions in other health dimensions remain difficult to quantify (as they often occur in the relationship and oneness perspectives), monetary costs have been calculated in some areas. For instance, we can consider how a heart problem in the physical health dimension and emotional problems in the psychological dimension generate productivity losses and economic costs for the American Dream. These examples highlight the extraordinary hidden costs suffered by the economy due to only two problems that occur in the other nine health dimensions.

Economic Costs of Heart Disease

Chronic diseases, such as cancer, diabetes, heart disease, pulmonary conditions, hypertension, and stroke, occur in the physical health dimension. The following example applies to only one of these conditions—heart disease. As the number one cause of death in the United States, heart disease haunts the population with its lethality. Survival of a heart attack often means that the person faces life-changing circumstances. For instance, depression and even post-traumatic stress disorder can accompany and negatively exacerbate the disease process (Edmonson, 2012). At least temporarily, the person is usually unable to perform as productively in her or his personal life, family, community, and employment setting. At the same time, extraordinary medical costs frequently accumulate.

When we consider the cumulative effects of heart disease on people throughout the United

States, the consequences are widespread and deleterious. Normally, we fail to recognize the direct and indirect effects that occur throughout society and often impact all the health dimensions. In this case, I will summarize direct and indirect economic costs identified and quantified that pertain only to losses in the workplace, though negative impacts to other dimensions are frequent and costly as well.

For instance, the projected direct treatment costs for heart disease in 2011 amounted to $101 billion (see Figure 6; Milken Institute, 2003a). However, if we initiate only moderate changes toward prevention and screening for heart disease, $12 billion in savings can be projected. Meanwhile, the estimated indirect costs accumulated from lost workdays and lower productivity for employees and their employed caregivers total $175 billion. Similarly, moderate changes in prevention and screening would save approximately $24 billion for heart disease alone that year.

When the baseline costs of heart disease are projected forward into 2023, the cumulative treatment costs throughout these years rise to $1.8 trillion. With moderate changes toward prevention and screening, the savings in treatment costs are projected at about $500 billion. The indirect costs accumulate to $3.1 trillion in lost productivity from 2011 through 2023. Similarly, moderate changes toward prevention and screening would save nearly $1 trillion over the period for this one chronic disease.

Economic Costs of Chronic Emotional Disorders

Although the economic costs of physical diseases are more frequently quantified, similar costs can be calculated in the psychological health dimension. For instance, chronic emotional disorders result in treatment costs projected at $69 billion and lost productivity costs at $282 billion in 2011 (see Figure 6, Milken Institute, 2003b). If moderate changes toward prevention and screening occurred, then $5 billion in treatment savings and $12 billion in lost productivity savings could be achieved in 2011. When projected into 2023, the treatment costs of emotional disorders accumulate to $1.3 trillion and the indirect costs accumulate to $5.3 trillion in lost productivity over these years. With moderate prevention and screening efforts, however, the savings in treatment costs could accrue to $200 billion and the lost productivity savings could accumulate to $500 billion.

Figure 6:
Projected Economic Costs of Heart Disease and Emotional Disorders

	2011	2023
Heart Disease		
Treatment Costs	$101 billion	$1.8 trillion
Prevention/screening savings	*$12 billion*	*$500 billion*
Lost Productivity	$175 billion	$3.1 trillion
Prevention/screening savings	*$24 billion*	*$1 trillion*
Emotional Disorders		
Treatment Costs	$69 billion	$1.3 trillion
Prevention/screening savings	*$5 billion*	*$200 billion*
Lost Productivity	$282 billion	$5.3 trillion
Prevention/screening savings	*$12 billion*	*$500 billion*
Total Costs		
Heart Disease + Emotional Disorders	$500 billion	$11.6 trillion
Prevention/screening savings	*$53 billion*	*$2.2 trillion*

Trillions of Dollars in Savings due to Prevention, Screening, and Healthy Living Practices

The economic and workplace costs to the American Dream due to only these two problem areas are enormous. In 2011, the treatment and lost productivity costs for heart disease and emotional disorders combined to total more than $500 billion. When these costs are projected from 2011 through 2023, the total costs for heart disease and emotional disorders soar to $11.6 trillion. Moderate changes toward prevention and screening for heart disease and emotional disorders could have accumulated $53 billion in savings in 2011 and amassed $2.2 trillion dollars in savings for the 2011–23 period.

Consequently, moderate efforts to prevent and screen for these two types of health problems could save trillions of dollars financially over time. Imagine the additional trillions of dollars that may be saved if we actually promoted healthy living among the general population that could prevent or at least delay the development of these two chronic conditions (see Bougsty, 2012, as well as the health care and education sections in chapter 7). Then imagine the additional trillions of dollars that we could likely save if we initiated moderate efforts to prevent and screen for problems throughout the twelve health dimensions listed earlier in the chapter. Finally, imagine the multiple trillions of dollars we could likely save if we intentionally promoted healthy living across the population to prevent and delay destructive conditions that range across the twelve health dimensions.

Healthy living appears to benefit the economy in significant other ways. For instance, improved health contributes not only to saving money but also to making money. Health improvements mean that we make more profits due to increased efficiency in the production of goods and services (Milken Institute, 2003c). A more productive and profitable economy typically means more opportunities, growth, and jobs for people.

Healthy Living Practices May Save the American Dream

If we simply teach and support people to implement the principles and practices of healthy living, we may do more to save the American Dream than anything else we can do. For example, healthy living supports increases in productivity and simultaneously supports decreases in the costs associated with dysfunctions that occur across the health spectrum. At the same time, healthy living supports us to grow, increase our creativity, develop resilience to sickness, and practice healthy lifestyles. These factors model and encourage the development of improved health throughout the population as well as the world.

As healthy living improves, we progressively shift the culture from relying predominantly on only three health dimensions, and instead, learn to utilize the full range of the twelve dimensions. In this way, we reduce the tendencies to continue developing problems, as we simultaneously promote improved functioning throughout our lives. If we then implement the healthy sustainable living practices described in chapters 9 and 10, we will work to enhance the sustainability of our health as well as the sustainability of our economic successes.

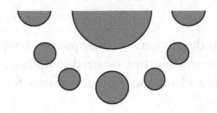

CHAPTER 6

A Universal Dream for Healthy Sustainable Living

● ● ● ● ● ● ● ● ●

Since all the health dimensions function in interdependent unity, a negative effect in one dimension naturally affects the other dimensions. For this reason, we can no longer afford to neglect or make nine of the health dimensions secondary to the three primary dimensions of the American Dream. If we continue to do so, we invite dysfunctions from secondary areas to undermine and threaten the American Dream, as well as threaten a healthy sustainable future.

We need a "Universal Dream for Healthy Sustainable Living" that values and balances all the health dimensions, so we can create a viable, successful future. This universal dream will transcend, yet include, the American Dream. For instance, the three major health dimensions affiliated with the American Dream fit naturally into the more comprehensive twelve dimensions of the universal dream. This new inclusive dream will protect the American Dream from the damages inflicted by dysfunctions in other dimensions, while providing a more comprehensive mission for the American Dream to serve. For example, we shift from a culture driven by money, power, and consumption to a cultural motivated by a healthy sustainable future and success for all.

The American Dream and the Capitalist Economic System Need to Serve this Universal Dream

Before examining how to create healthy sustainable living, we need to understand how our existing institutions inadvertently undermine our efforts to achieve this goal. For instance, while the American Dream tends to neglect nine of the twelve dimensions necessary for healthy living, it also operates on several outdated assumptions that can harm our future as described in the following sections. Many of these assumptions derive from the capitalist economic system that largely underlies the American Dream.

These economic assumptions and their consequences influence different societal institutions, such as our political democratic system, our media, health care, and education systems, as will be described in chapter 7. While we have achieved major economic and technological successes by acting on these assumptions, devolutionary consequences have also been accumulating that we can no longer afford to ignore. At this time we need to update and evolve these old economic assumptions so they align with and support this new vision for health and sustainability for humanity and the planet.

Capitalism Needs to Evolve to Create a Healthy Sustainable Future

In the United States, the capitalist economic system emerged several centuries ago and has guided the development of the country's vast natural and human resources. The economic system has proven so successful that most of the global community has now adapted some version of the system to lead us into the future. Nevertheless, several features of the capitalist system must evolve in order to overcome the threats they introduce to us and the world.

The development of healthy sustainable living depends upon our willingness to evolve the capitalist economic system. Six specific limitations built into the system will be highlighted here. In Figure 7, each limitation will be paired with a positive solution that describes how to evolve capitalism to support health and sustainability. In this way, we can update the economic system and, at the same time, incorporate the American Dream into a universal dream that challenges us to develop a successful future for all humanity and the planet.

Present Value: Money

The first fundamental limitation associated with capitalism involves the lack of value assigned to crucial components of *reality*. Without accurately valuing all the vital aspects of the world, we lack the necessary information to live harmoniously with the whole. For instance, the capitalist system normally relies upon money to define value. Along these lines, the assignment of monetary value to material goods and services (generally consistent with the separateness perspective) works quite well. Nevertheless, a living person or a whole living system that operates significantly from the relationship and oneness perspectives cannot be easily assigned monetary values. Therefore, economic decision making that significantly runs the country and the world must include all the variables that contribute value in *reality*, and not merely the ones easily given monetary value.

The Foundations of Capitalism Are Viewed as Externalities

The two variables that create and run our economic system—people and the planet—inherently have value. The economic system, however, can only minimally measure this value as it quantifies such aspects as human labor and productivity, as well as quantifies natural resources as they become commodities. Since people and the planet typically function in complex relationships and perform as whole systems, the economy struggles to place monetary value on these critical operations in the relationship and oneness realms of *reality*. Therefore, the people who provide the essential human resources and the planet that supplies the necessary natural resources for the economy to exist, as well as function, are often seen as externalities—lacking quantifiable value in a capitalist society.

Figure 7:
The Evolution of Capitalism to Serve Healthy Sustainable Living

Capitalism	Healthy Sustainable Living
Value: Money	Ethics of Healthy Sustainable Living + Money
Process: Dependence on Material Reality & Money primarily	Win-Win Relationships shift Separateness to Oneness via Love + Money
Goal: Growth through Material consumption primarily	Growth through Information consumption & expanded Spiritual awareness + Material consumption
Motivation: Competition primarily	Cooperation and Trust prioritized
Rights: Separate, individual & corporate, special interests	Collective, public & planetary interests balanced & prioritized relative to Separate special interests
Power: Authoritarian & authoritative	Democratic & authoritative

Figure 8:
Three Perspectives of Reality Relative to Capitalism Compared to Healthy Sustainable Living

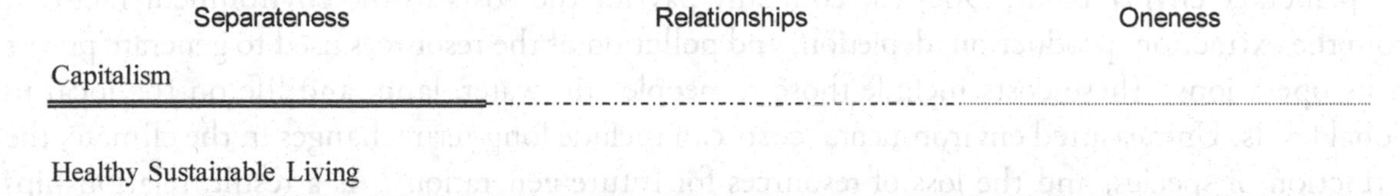

Separateness	Relationships	Oneness
Capitalism		
Healthy Sustainable Living		

As a result, the evolutionary value embedded in people and the planet has become less important than the commercial value of products and services. We have created an economic system in which we frequently learn to value human creations over actual human beings, as well as over nature itself. Since the economy depends upon people and the environment for its ultimate existence, we have created a partial and, in the end, a self-destructive value system. We perceive the portions of *reality* that we prefer or we find convenient to measure. Meanwhile, we often neglect or fail to perceive and value the world fully enough to create a sustainable future.

Furthermore, the system places monetary value largely on material objects, reflective of the separateness lens. Subsequently, the system significantly fails to value the relationships and oneness lenses. Consequently, the lack of value for significant aspects of *reality*, accompanied by the externalization of human and environmental costs and benefits to the world, produces an unsustainable system, as currently conceived. Unless we evolve the capitalist economy to value people, the planet, and all *reality* as essential for its existence we appear on an unsustainable path.

Externalities can be beneficial or negative. As an example, when a company terminates an employee, it may subsequently recognize the beneficial externality that the employee provided in terms of human relationships. Such relationships may include those within the company, but also with consumers, outside agencies, the media, and the larger society. Although the employee may be easy to replace, the hidden value and information shared in all these relationships often takes years to regain.

In contrast, an example of a negative externality involves the company's relationships with the planetary environment. Does the company pay for the costs to the environment incurred from the extraction, production, depletion, and pollution of the resources used to generate profits in its operations? These costs include those to people, air, water, land, and life on the local to global levels. Unmeasured environmental costs can include long-term changes in the climate, the extinction of species, and the loss of resources for future generations. As a result, relationships with people and the planet often accrue enormous costs beyond the monetary values assigned by the present capitalist system and, therefore, represent negative externalities.

Future Value: Ethics of Healthy Sustainable Living + Money

An ethical system based on healthy sustainable living provides methods to value *reality* more fully and accurately, as presented in chapter 9. Our current economy needs to evolve to overcome its seemingly lethal limitations that substantially neglect to value the people and the planet upon which the system exists. In addition, the economy needs to operate consistent with all three lenses—the separateness, relationships, and oneness perspectives—necessary for us to perceive and live harmoniously with *reality*.

The proposed ethical system helps us overcome these fatal flaws. First, the ethical model portrays a comprehensive overview of *reality*. This provides a picture of all the health dimensions across all the major levels of human life, as well as all the major levels of planetary evolution. In other words, it provides a means to value people and the planet and prevent harm to both. Then the model provides a triple-lens view of the separate health dimensions as they interact in relationships across all levels of society and the world as a whole.

From these comprehensive perspectives we can consider how any action that we initiate reverberates through the complex relationships that connect the economic activity to potential outcomes in human society and in the planetary environment. We can also take both a short- and a long-term perspective of the consequences, such as described in chapter 9. In this way, we can go beyond our normal planning efforts to consider the long-term evolutionary and devolutionary outcomes of any action. As an example, a nuclear power plant may provide a variety of short-term and a few long-term benefits, but ultimately, it produces toxic radiation that can persist longer than human civilization has even existed.

The ethical living model introduces a single, relatively simple model to help analyze the potential positive and negative consequences of any action. This ethical perspective will support decision making to achieve short- and long-term success. It encourages actions that contribute to evolution and prevents actions that introduce devolutionary threats to our lives. Therefore, evolution versus devolution emerges as the ultimate ethical criteria for decision making. This contrasts with the present decision making process in which money and short-term profits tend to dominate our business and societal choices.

A transcend-and-include methodology applies to the present capitalist economic system. The ultimate purpose for creating a healthy sustainable future for humanity transcends yet can include the functions and many goals of the economic system. Hence, we need to evolve the economy into service to this larger vision. As an example, the use of money and the principles of the American Dream of success will continue as long as they support the larger mission. The ethics for a viable future takes precedence over and is served by the continued use of money, whenever appropriate. Decision making shifts to value healthy sustainable living as primary, with money serving it secondarily. This means that we align with human evolution and value human life as the priority; the artificial life of the economy, although very important, becomes secondary. It continues to function as a creative production of human life.

The ethical living model provides a means to consider the complex human and planetary features of *reality* and their interdependent relationships. We can then minimize the chances to overlook important variables and consequences that may otherwise undermine our future viability. The model serves as a guide for us to create evolutionary growth, while we simultaneously avoid devolutionary destruction throughout the world. (See chapter 9 for an application of the ethical living model to the complex issue of fossil fuel use, so we can analyze both the evolutionary and devolutionary potential outcomes in relation to the universal goal for healthy sustainable living.)

Present Process: Dependence on Material Reality and Money Primarily

The capitalist economic system emerged predominantly during the Industrial Age. It faced particular challenges to modify and engage in the development of nature and the material world. Consequently, the relationship and oneness perspectives received minimal attention during the development and progression of the economic system. Instead, the economy depended largely upon material reality to function and produce success. In addition, money measured value within the system and objectified that value through the use of material objects, such as coins, bills, and quantitative figures. Thus, the economic system continues to depend predominantly on material reality, including its material means of measuring value.

As a result, our evolutionary predisposition, in which we perceive material reality and separateness as primary, has been strongly reinforced by the capitalist economy. We perceive the separate objects of money and consumer goods as possessing value. Therefore, we normally want to connect with these items. Recall that as evolution proceeds, separate objects function in relationships to form more complex, organized wholes. Thus, as participants in evolution, we naturally want our separateness to function in relationships with other objects, especially those with perceived value, so we can interact and create a greater sense of oneness and wholeness.

For example, we consume or attach to new clothes, a car, a house, or a cell phone that frequently gives a temporary sense that it belongs to us, thereby expanding our identity. When we connect our separateness via relationships into a sense of oneness, such as when the cell phone feels like a part of us, we often experience feelings of pleasure, happiness, and fulfillment. Sometimes we can even experience a brief spiritual awakening in which we suddenly realize our deeper, inherent oneness with *reality*. For instance, if we awaken to *reality* in a new way, we may experience an inspirational "aha" moment. Initially, we may connect with a sense of oneness with the object or the situation that we perceive. In this process, we may activate a brief spiritual awakening in which we experience the joy of oneness with *reality* that prevails beyond our prior realizations.

Dependencies or Addictions to Money and Consumption Can Develop

When we attach to a valuable object to improve our life and we experience happiness and potentially a brief spiritual sense of oneness, we tend to want to repeat the experience. When money or material goods generate such positive outcomes, we may decide to earn more money or purchase on credit in order to consume more of the goods. Since the pleasures generated by these connections usually last only a short time, we have to repeat the behaviors to continue the pleasure. In the process, habitual patterns of attraction and seeking may develop that eventually convert into dependencies. In some cases, the habitual pursuit of money and the consumption of material goods provide immediate pleasure but can also lead to personal harm or damage to other people and the world. In these cases, an addiction develops in which the habitual behavior is accompanied by harmful results.

Beyond the pleasure that often motivates people in dependencies and addictions, negative feelings and experiences can also motivate these habitual patterns. For example, when we lose our temporary high after a connection with a paycheck or a consumer purchase, we tend to slip back into perceptions of separateness. In the context of the universe, we may feel small and isolated or even experience a sense of emptiness and meaninglessness. In an effort to escape isolated, empty feelings or replace other negative feelings, we may consume additional goods and services. In this way, we temporarily feel more connected and full again.

These habitual patterns may provide immediate pleasure or relieve personal distress. Yet they usually distract us from the growth required to perceive more accurate, full views of *reality*. These habits can then trap us in the perspective of separateness that restricts our potential to expand our consciousness. Furthermore, when we focus primarily on the separateness lens of the three perspectives of *reality*, we increase the risks of damaging the relationships and the whole systems that support our lives. Ultimately, our capacities to achieve healthy sustainable living require overcoming such dependencies. Otherwise, they restrict our awareness and our choices regarding how to live in harmony with the world.

Future Process: Win-Win Relationships Shift Separateness to Oneness via Love + Money

Love can be conceptualized beyond its traditional romantic version. In this case, love represents the relationship process in which separate participants engage in give-and-take exchanges for mutual, win-win benefits that lead to more effective, whole functioning. Thus, love converts our normal sense of separateness into interconnected relationships that contribute to our personal and interdependent oneness. In this way, love integrates all three perspectives of *reality*. Ultimately, love serves as the core dynamic in evolution that transforms the universe from separateness into relationships that form greater oneness (see chapter 10). In these ways, love enlivens the world and provides a key to our future conscious evolution.

The economy successfully employs a limited form of this love as producers and consumers mutually exchange goods and services for win-win gains. The producer wins in selling products and making a profit, while consumers win in purchasing desired goods and services. This win-win arrangement represents a limited form of love restricted to the special interests involved. This special interest love reveals a positive feature in the economy that we can retain, but will need to expand in order to promote healthy sustainable living.

For instance, love in economic exchanges can ideally expand to encompass a win-win-win-win-win approach in which producers, consumers, humanity, the planet, and evolution all win. In this way, love for the participants will experience greater breadth and substantially more meaning as it benefits the collective interests of all affected by the action. Accordingly, our economic system can promote the processes of evolution, as producers and consumers benefit not only themselves but also the rest of *reality*.

To propagate the evolutionary nature of love, we need to exchange goods and services in winning relationships that also enhance trust and a sense of oneness for all involved. In these ways, we can contribute to human progress in evolution. Nonetheless, money functions as an intervening variable in this process. Since money usually takes the form of a material object that artificially represents value, we often give it more attention and valence than we give love. Instead of the natural flow and inherent value of the loving process guiding our economic behaviors, material outcomes typically guide our actions. Since both capitalism and our brain function with a predisposition to perceive material reality, money and material consumption usually attract more attention than love.

To counteract this tendency, we need to affirm love as the primary dynamic necessary to guide our exchanges in the economy, similar to its role in evolution. In this context, love refers to the relationship process in which separate participants engage in give-and-take exchanges for mutual win-win benefits that lead to more effective whole functioning. The conscious experience of love in any economic exchange needs to be prioritized, as the exchange represents more than the goods and services exchanged. It represents evolution in action. The material exchange is accompanied by relationship exchanges that can generate a greater sense of connection, trust, happiness, and oneness.

We cocreate slightly new realities with each winning exchange; these exchanges transform portions of *reality* from separateness into relationships toward oneness. Thus, we can experience our deeper evolutionary nature as we consciously experience the loving process involved in our everyday economic exchanges.

We can still use money to facilitate exchanges, but we can add value to the transaction by experiencing the love involved in the process. Capitalism can, therefore, evolve with money as the practical means for material exchanges, while love functions as the conscious process in the relationship exchanges. Both material and relationship exchanges occur in any economic transaction, but our challenge involves how to make the relationship exchange consciously more important and enduring than the material exchange. The relationship is ultimately more important because it can continue to grow, while in contrast, the material object naturally decays.

As an example, when we purchase a lunch from a food vendor, we exchange money for the material food. At the same time we exchange information regarding the relationship between the vendor and ourselves, ranging from happiness to indifference to anger. Although the food will be consumed and require further material exchanges for additional consumption, the relationship between the vendor and us has the capacity to evolve and grow. The relationship will most likely grow towards greater cooperation and shared oneness through intentionally communicating in loving manners that acknowledge and appreciate the value the vendor adds to our lives in these material and relationship exchanges. Consequently, the food provides physical nourishment, while the relationship can evolve to provide emotional, social, and spiritual nourishment. Future purchases exchange similar quantities of money, while the relationship can increase qualitatively in a variety of important ways.

Ultimately, the loving exchanges in win-win-win-win-win relationships will also prove more important, as these exchanges encourage further growth, embracing self- and collective interests. From the personal standpoint, we can enjoy the practice of love as we experience greater meaning and happiness. From the collective standpoint, the practice of love leads to increased safety and trust among the participants that invites further participation in growth opportunities. From the evolutionary perspective the process of love functions at the core of healthy sustainable living, as each exchange attempts to benefit all.

Present Goal: Growth through Material Consumption

A basic assumption within the capitalist economic system involves the need for growth. In general, this assumption parallels evolutionary processes. Historically, however, such growth has occurred largely through the consumption of material goods and services. Since the material resources for such growth are limited by the finite nature of the planet, we cannot grow endlessly dependent on material consumption alone. Furthermore, consumption of material objects invites us to focus on the object and neglect our interconnected relationships and our oneness with *reality* overall.

Hence, growth through material consumption often leads to the depletion of natural resources (for example, fresh water, rare earth minerals, and fossil fuels), as well as to pollution with material byproducts that disrupt the existing relationships between resources and the ecosystems on the planet. As resources diminish, discovering new ones will typically become more expensive and frequently more destructive to the environment. Conflicts will likely develop between corporate and national competitors. These disruptions will tend to undermine our long-term health and sustainability.

Future Goal: Growth through Information Consumption and Expanded Spiritual Awareness + Material Consumption

Information consumption represents the emerging stage of capitalist development. Cell phones and the Internet provide accelerating access to the exponentially growing volumes of information being created throughout the world. Information appears infinite and avoids many of the harmful side effects often associated with material consumption. Material resources tend to be finite, breakdown, and pollute. Therefore, information consumption increasingly needs to replace material consumption, especially once basic material needs are met. We will need to continue to develop alternatives for growing the economy with information consumption that will likely minimize harm to people and the planet in comparison to most material consumption.

Beyond material and information consumption, we also need to expand our capabilities to gain spiritual awareness. We can gain such awareness through traditional practices such as meditation, contemplation, and prayer. Yet, we can also initiate subtle spiritual awakenings any time we integrate the three perspectives of *reality*. For instance, when we expand our awareness from the separateness perspective and experience our natural connections with others and the world, we can suddenly realize our oneness with all within our awareness. In other words, we can awaken to our separate and interconnected human natures, in the context of our inherent oneness with *reality*. Thus, we directly experience our ever-present spiritual nature when we awaken to our oneness with all. More subtly, we experience what might be called miniature spiritual awakenings whenever we experience our oneness with a person, object, or process within *reality*.

As we expand our consumption of information and awaken to our spiritual nature, we evolve our consciousness to perceive *reality* more fully. Expanded awareness of information tends to awaken the relationship lens, while spiritual realizations open the oneness lens. Thus, we increasingly expand and integrate our perceptions through the use of all three lenses. These forms of increased consciousness further open the door to develop healthy sustainable living.

As we perceive more fully and accurately, we can consciously choose how to create benefits and avoid harm. We can initiate actions that contribute to others, the planet, evolution, and all *reality* simultaneously as we also prevent any significant harm. Consequently, expansions in our consciousness should rise to the top of the priority list for our future growth. Through greater awareness, we can progressively transform our lives and the economy to function in increasing integrity with *reality*.

Present Motivation: Competition primarily

Capitalism relies largely on competition to stimulate growth. Common knowledge holds that competition drives the economy, represents the engine of growth, keeps prices down, and encourages innovation and efficiency (Bougsty-Marshall, 2012). Competitively striving to produce the best for less has proven extraordinarily successful for consumers and the economy. From the economic perspective, all these assertions have credence.

Nevertheless, when we expand our perceptions and value system to the perspective of healthy sustainable living that aligns more fully and accurately with *reality*, we gain additional insights. While the conclusions about competition appear true from the limited economic perspective, the benefits associated with competition also have costs.

In some cases, the costs appear to lead toward devolutionary consequences, especially when we rely too heavily on competition. For instance, competition arises primarily from the egocentric and ethnocentric perspectives of special interests. Since they perceive only limited portions of *reality*, they will eventually produce unsustainable conditions. For example, while special interests may succeed in the short run, they often stimulate harm in areas beyond their immediate concerns. For instance, material goods generally derive from finite material resources that slowly suffer depletion and often generate pollution that undermine health and sustainability. Furthermore, competition can drive down prices, but sometimes at the expense of employees as their incomes do not increase commensurate with the amount of work or with the cost of living.

The cost savings that result from competition can come from technological advances or increased efficiencies but too often come from using or exploiting people and the planet as they appear as externalities. With limited monetary value attached and accompanied by limited accountability, people and the planet can suffer damages. Such competitive actions then add to the numerous local, national, and global problems among people and nations, as well as to the damages inflicted on the air, water, and land environments of the planet that support our lives.

Competition arises from the separateness lens. In a world of complex, interdependent relationships that have to function as a whole for life to continue, the separateness perspective is unsustainable if used exclusively. It too often exploits the whole in efforts to satisfy its special interests. For instance, the human and environmental problems contributed to by competitive actions appear through the separateness lens as problems external to us. These problems do not directly appear to affect our special interest concerns.

Nevertheless, perceived through the relationship and oneness lenses, these problems suddenly become personal due to our interconnected relationships and our interdependent oneness with these dangers. In this more accurate and inclusive version of the situation, we realize both the benefits and the costs. While competition has its benefits, it can simultaneously threaten others and the world. We begin to appreciate that these threats can eventually affect us.

Furthermore, each individual or special interest group engages in competition in an effort to win. Thus, competition promotes win-lose relationships. The winner in a capitalist system often receives money, accolades for success, and further opportunities, while the losers suffer. These rewards from winning frequently dominate our attention and take priority over participating in the next necessary step in evolution—cooperation.

In the case of the winner, cooperation may occur in a limited, special interest way. For instance, a corporation will likely direct its personnel to cooperate in efforts to produce and sell the winning product. This special interest orientation, however, fails to cooperate beyond the corporation. Therefore, the creative ideas present among the various competitors generally fail to integrate into more comprehensive, advanced innovations that could further benefit society and the world.

In such a win-lose context, when participants lose, instead of promoting cooperation and oneness as consistent with evolution, increased separateness usually occurs. Thus, one step forward in innovations toward greater oneness is accompanied by at least one step backward as relationships devolve into separateness. As a result, competition often reduces the desire to cooperate and, thereby, serves to restrict potentials for further growth and evolution.

In addition, the trust necessary to support future cooperation also suffers. Since competition leaves us continuously vulnerable to the threat of loss, trust can further erode from chronic fear. When trust is directly damaged by an intentional violation during a competitive struggle, it is normally difficult to regain. For instance, when a competitor uses unfair practices to win, this tends to stimulate fear, anger, and revenge, which further undermines the potentials to regain trust and develop a cooperative relationship. When competition results in violence, for instance, trust can be violated to such degrees that people refuse to trust again, leading to intractable conflicts.

In these ways, competition tends to undermine cooperation. Competition also undermines the trust necessary for effective functioning in relationships (for instance, in marriages, families, organizations, businesses, communities, and nations). Competition that fails to progress into cooperation also impedes progress in evolution, as well as precludes the development of a productive, sustainable economy and society.

Future Motivation: Cooperation and Trust Prioritized

Capitalism needs to follow the lead of evolution. Since competition occurs as an early to middle step in the creative process of change (see figures 1–3), it represents an important yet insufficient aspect of sustainable growth. The necessary next step requires participants to work together in cooperation, ideally using conscious, loving exchanges that intentionally create win-win outcomes in which all participants benefit. Growth can then continue by building the trust necessary for long-term relationships to support further cooperation and innovation. Trust naturally increases and frees participants to expand their consciousness, creativity, and willingness to shift competition into constructive cooperation that can accelerate growth toward benefiting the whole. The later evolutionary steps can then follow to increase the organization, order, and oneness of the new creation.

Cooperation epitomizes a fundamental step for our economic and societal development, as well as an essential step toward functioning in congruence with evolution. No wonder the happiest countries in the world tend to integrate economic growth in the context of cooperation, equality, trust, and representative governance (Helliwell, Layard, and Sachs, 2012). As the economy follows the processes of evolution, we naturally accelerate our progress toward healthy sustainable living.

Present Rights: Separate, Individual and Corporate, Special interests

Capitalism tends to treat material reality perceived through the separateness lens as *reality*. Consistent with these views, separate individuals and corporations enjoy special powers in the economy. For instance, individuals and corporations receive special interest rights that frequently prioritize their functioning over public and planetary interests.

In a sense, the capitalist system portrays corporations and even the economic system itself with what might be called "artificial life." Although a corporation and the economy are not alive biologically, we sometimes treat them like they are alive. For instance, both the economy and corporations require ongoing growth and profits to feed their functions and preserve their existence. Sometimes, they even need to be rescued from failure and death because so many employees, the society, and the world community depend on their existence. Accordingly, the capitalist system and its individual and corporate players have gained profound powers.

The economy and its players need to grow and make profits. Quantitative measures and monetary values have been developed to demonstrate the growth and profit profiles, as well as other associated needs related to the survival and success of the economy and corporations.

In contrast, the interests and needs of people and the planetary environment have minimal quantifiable measures to delineate what they need to survive and thrive.

Consequently, the capitalist economy and its affiliated corporate and individual interests normally win when they compete with the collective interests of humanity and the planet. The artificial life of the economy and the corporations typically prevails as more important, or more justifiable, than the unquantifiable needs of real human beings, the planetary environment, and evolutionary processes. Ironically, we engender the economy and corporations with artificial lives and then often prioritize these artificial lives as more important and valuable than our actual human lives. As a result, the capitalist system, corporations, and individuals continue to gain rights and special interest benefits. Meanwhile, the health and sustainability concerns relative to people, the planet, and evolutionary processes remain largely in the background. When life and evolutionary systems reside in the background, they can be innocently or intentionally exploited to feed the profit and growth needs of special interest individuals, corporations, and national economies.

While the economy and corporations have the need to grow, their incentive to make a profit drives them to earn more money. Too often, the profits are prioritized as more important than meeting the real needs of people and the planet's environments. For instance, billions of people in the world suffer, and many millions die, from the lack of clean water, adequate food, sanitation, and sufficient health care. Yet the profit incentive in the capitalist system invites corporations to market and sell goods and services that satisfy mostly the desires and preferences of more affluent consumers. In the process, they often ignore many of the genuine human needs that exist throughout the world. Thus, an unsuspecting bias toward the development of a world of haves and have-nots occurs. In the end, the capitalist economy and its corporations often serve their special interests and artificial lives as more important than human lives and the living systems of the planetary environment.

Future Rights: Collective Public and Planetary Interests Balanced and Prioritized Relative to Separate Special interests

Collective interests generally reside in the background beyond the rights, freedoms, and powers available to individuals, corporations, and the national and global economic systems. Since humans and the planet provide the essential resources and relationships necessary for the economy, corporations, and other special interests to exist, the common interests of humanity and the planet need placed in the foreground. In order to seek a sustainable future, the collective public and planetary interests need to be prioritized. Only when these common interests survive can the economy survive or, for that matter, can we survive.

Special interests generally represent limited, more short-term concerns while common interests more often represent comprehensive, long-term sustainability concerns. By understanding special interests and collective interests across the planet, we can better comprehend how to balance their competing and cooperative needs. Healthy sustainable living provides a comprehensive value system from which to analyze and prescribe solutions to balance these diverse concerns. When in doubt, the collective interests need to be prioritized. The planetary support systems and humanity as a whole have to function and survive for special interests to prevail.

Present Power: Authoritarian and Authoritative

The power structure applied originally in the capitalist system generally involved an authoritarian style in which the owner or boss controlled the enterprise. Strict obedience to the dictatorial powers of the boss was generally expected and enforced. Since they owned the business, they acted in the role of the owner and the employees performed more like cogs in the enterprise. In general, money served as the carrot to motivate employees and the threat of job loss served as the stick. This top-down power to direct others to work for the company represented a "Win-win" relationship at times (where the boss enjoyed the big Win versus the employees' smaller win) but turned into a "Win-lose" relationship whenever employees suffered from exploitation. Such relationships, based on unequal power, often led to significant discrepancies in pay and eventually contributed to the problems of the haves and have-nots.

As employees organized through groups and unions, their collective power appeared to threaten authoritarian employers with the potential of a lose-win relationship. Therefore, more cooperative Win-win agreements started to emerge. This helped shift the power structure from the traditional authoritarian dominance toward authoritative rule. In general, an authoritative style of power involves executives or bosses who have the authority and power to make decisions and direct employee work. Ideally, these authorities respect the input of their employees regarding decisions and practices creating a top-down and bottom-up approach. The hierarchical structure involved with authoritative power often provides guidelines for information sharing, decision making, income determination, and power within the company, so employees experience more Win-win relationships.

Future Power: Democratic and Authoritative

The natural model for power and success in the business world comes from the processes of evolution (see figures 1–3). In this case, we can examine and apply successes tested over millions of years in evolution to help businesses and capitalism succeed. Since businesses already operate within these natural dynamics of evolution, they can simply become aware and then start practicing these basic evolutionary principles to improve their business success.

For example, from the perspective of evolution, authoritative decision making improves upon authoritarian power structures in most cases. From the authoritative viewpoint, growth processes can be enhanced when bosses appreciate the unique creativity of employees. Both the perceptions and the actions of employees contribute to the diversity of possibilities that could introduce positive change into the business operations. By listening to and incorporating ideas and actions from employees, executives can further improve the effectiveness and efficiencies of production and sales. In contrast, authoritarian rule usually relies on the limited consciousness and creativity of only one person—the boss.

Nevertheless, sustainable business practices depend significantly upon the next important step in evolution—cooperation. Recall that conscious evolution proceeds in the direction of increasing consciousness, creativity, competition, cooperation, organization, order, and into greater complexity and oneness. To maximize our opportunities for sustainable change, therefore, we need as many different perspectives and potential actions as possible. These can be provided through democratic processes in which everyone shares and competes initially with their unique consciousness and actions.

Ideally, democratic processes then invite cooperation to organize and order the diverse inputs into more complex, unified choices for change. From an evolutionary perspective then, democracy appears as our best hope for future decision making in businesses, as well as in most settings throughout the world. An exception may apply to urgent decisions that may need to employ increasingly streamlined versions of democratic rule. If an agreement cannot be formed, an authoritative decision making process may be necessary.

Democratic Processes in the Workplace Can Parallel Evolutionary Processes

The growth process generally proceeds as follows: Democracy welcomes the unique perceptions (consciousness) of all the participants in order to consider the different viewpoints (competition; see figure 2). Each perception typically contains some aspects of the truth of the larger whole. As people progressively understand the various facets of the situation, cooperation can generate further creativity to help organize these distinct perceptions into greater complexity and order. When sufficient agreement occurs regarding how to synthesize the multiplicity of views (unity or oneness), then we can choose actions to introduce changes into the world. Thus, democratic decision making enables us to cocreate with information in *reality* by consciously following the natural processes upon which evolution succeeds.

Metaphorically, if we consider *reality* as a puzzle, the more pieces of the whole that we perceive, the more we tend to understand. With sufficient understanding, we can choose actions that place our situation into alignment with the larger *reality*. As we align our piece of the puzzle to fit into the larger whole, we move toward creating a more sustainable future.

In this context, authoritative views are natural and necessary but typically represent only limited pieces of the whole puzzle. Authoritative special interest perceptions are usually too limited to understand the whole and are, consequently, too limited to create sustainable change.

When democratic processes are employed, the perception of each individual counts. These perceptions may add unique pieces to the puzzle, or they may collaborate with other views to reinforce certain parts of the puzzle. Ideally, the differences and commonalities can be synthesized into agreements among the participants. In combination the individual and collective pieces produce a more complete picture of the situation. As the puzzle emerges to reveal mutual understanding, actions can be democratically chosen to integrate the special interests of the participants with the collective interests of the society and the environment. As a consequence, the capitalist economic system can increasingly support the evolution of authoritarian to authoritative to democratic decision making processes. In the process, we can accelerate our advances toward a healthy sustainable future.

In addition, employees can be motivated to contribute passionately at work by providing them more equitable pay. Since all work is work, more equitable distribution of benefits can create more Win-Win relationships. Providing employees with opportunities to own stock or take ownership in the business may significantly increase productivity, morale, commitment, profit sharing, and working for the good of the whole. In addition, mutual ownership, profit sharing, and equitable pay could help reduce the inequities experienced between the haves and the have-nots. Democracy in the workplace also encourages individuals to shift from their perceptions of separateness and increasingly perceive their interconnected relationships and interdependent oneness with others and the world. These perceptual shifts promoted by democratic rule significantly advance our abilities to contribute to the development of healthy sustainable corporations that support a viable future for all.

Overview: The Need to Evolve Our Capitalist Economic System

A healthy sustainable future depends upon comprehending and living in harmony with *reality*. Therefore, any personal, corporate, and national actions that fail to align with the world as a whole may present threats to our future. Thus, the capitalist system grows based on the apparent assumptions that special interests and short-term profits will lead to collective, long-term, human and planetary well-being and sustainability. Yet, self-interests frequently gain at the expense of collective interests. When the relationship and oneness perspectives suffer due to an overemphasis on the separateness perspective, as promoted by the capitalist system, devolution rather than evolution will likely prevail (see Figure 3).

The present capitalist system provides an inadequate means of comprehending and integrating the three perspectives of *reality* necessary to develop healthy sustainable living (see Figure 8 portrayed earlier with Figure 7). The capitalist system focuses primarily on the separateness perspective, much less so on the relationship viewpoint, and minimally on the oneness perspective. In contrast, healthy sustainable living values and integrates all three perspectives as necessary to generate more accurate, full perceptions of *reality*.

Profits can quickly become an end in themselves. All the participants—consumers, producers, and the economy itself—depend on adequate finances. Money symbolically becomes the lifeblood that motivates most of the participants. In other words, profits depict value, measured by money, which can convert into material goods and services. The participants can then become dependent, if not addicted to money and material goods and services. In the short-run, corporations and the economy generally benefit from high demands for money and consumption. Eventually, however, the short-term success can turn into long-term impairment of the populace and the planet (for example, through exploitation and pollution) that then threatens the corporations and the economy.

The Capitalist Economy Needs to Operate in Service to Healthy Sustainable Living

If we intend to overcome the problems we have created in the world, the capitalist system needs to envision and implement a higher purpose than growth and profits to create a viable future for all. In addition, if we want the economic system itself to survive, it needs to align with the processes of evolution. Therefore, capitalism needs to evolve to value all people and the environments of the planet. Moreover, the interdependent relationships that occur among people, the planet, and profits need to support healthy sustainable living. The system also will have to shift from material consumption toward information consumption and the development of spiritual awareness as new priorities. These shifts promote expanded consciousness.

For sustainable growth the economy needs to follow the natural processes of evolution. The universe evolves by separate entities engaging in give-and-take exchanges in relationships that move toward the development of oneness on a higher order of more complex functioning. In other words, love represents the process in which evolution moves from separateness through relationships into oneness that evolves the universe.

Relative to our current economic system, love begins to emerge when people share in give-and-take exchanges for mutual benefits that generate growth and invites movement toward greater oneness. Nonetheless, people typically focus on the exchange from the separateness perspective in which goods and services appear as the benefit to one party and money appears as the value to the other party. The underlying loving process in the exchange needs to be consciously experienced in order to shift from a special interest event into a relationship win for all the participants—the consumer, producer, humanity, the planet, and evolution.

Consciousness of the loving process involved in economic exchanges means that unique creativity and competition represent only preliminary steps. Sustainable growth depends on increases in cooperation to create more organization and order that integrate into complex wholes. The separateness perspective among people and objects needs to expand to value all the interconnected relationships involved. The potential then emerges to create greater oneness of evolved functioning that contributes to health, happiness, and sustainability.

Capitalism, based primarily on private special interests, may maximize growth but often does so by accompanying destruction that undermines the sustainability of the whole. For instance, it draws resources from the larger wholes of humanity and the environment, as if these two foundations of life can be exploited forever to serve the special interests of individuals, corporations, nations, and the economic system.

Separate individuals, corporations, and nations compete for their special interests but often unknowingly exploit the collective interests of the whole. Apparently, the assumption is that satisfying the special interests will also satisfy the collective interests. Unfortunately, rapid growth of these special interests can also occur at the expense of the overall system. When the special interests gain priority over collective interests, destruction can occur to the collective.

In this way, capitalism sometimes resembles a cancer. Similarly, cancer can demonstrate remarkable growth, but in the process destroys its host as well as itself. A major difference between a cancer and our special interest growth is that we can consciously recognize and transcend the destructive risks of our special interest nature. We can intentionally promote personal, group, human, planetary, and evolutionary health and sustainability for all as the cure.

We now need to evolve the capitalist economic system to function in greater integrity with *reality*. The current system operates based on at least the six assumptions presented here that portend unsustainable outcomes. This means that we need to develop a system of values that transcends the limited capitalist values yet includes the successful components of the system that have brought us so far. For instance, we may continue to use money but do so in service to the higher values to create win-win-win-win-win relationships that increase cooperation, trust, and love. Special interest gratification and monetary profits continue as long as they also support collective interests and generate no significant harm. Cooperative information growth, spiritual awakenings, democratic participation, and increased consciousness need prioritized, so we can evolve the capitalist economy to function in alignment with the ethics of healthy sustainable living.

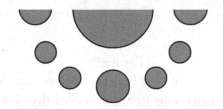

CHAPTER 7

The Evolution of Societal Institutions to Create a Healthy Sustainable Future

● ● ● ● ● ● ●

Along with capitalism, other societal institutions need to evolve if we want to create a healthy sustainable future. Our institutions shape and reinforce how we perceive and act in our lives. At the same time, they affect the evolution or devolution of our future. As examples, the following four institutions need to evolve to support healthy sustainable living:

1. Political—democracy;

2. Media;

3. Health care; and

4. Education (see Figure 9).

Each institution has its own history, assumptions that guide its functioning, and values regarding its purposes in serving the public. A brief example of how the capitalist system competes with and often compromises the functioning of these institutions and their services follows. While money defines value in the capitalist system, money also defines value in these institutions. Yet the value of money often competes with the values of the services that the institutions offer.

Unfortunately, diminished services from these societal institutions can result in deficiencies in service delivery to the public and sometimes lead to devolutionary changes instead of evolutionary growth. An example will be presented for each institution related to how the influence of the present capitalist values can limit the evolutionary potentials of their services. Recommendations will then be provided on how to solve these dysfunctions, so each institution can more productively evolve, help the capitalist system evolve, and ultimately support the development of a healthy sustainable future.

Figure 9:
Proposals for the Evolution of Our Political Democracy, Media, Health Care,
and Education Institutions to Support Healthy Sustainable Living

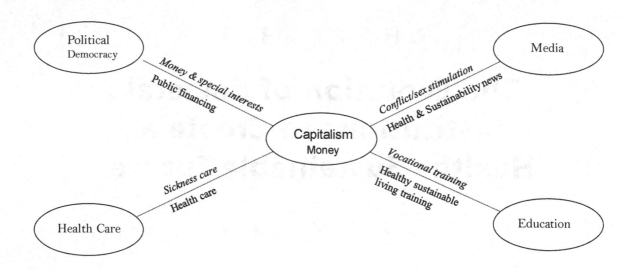

Political—Democracy

The United States implemented democracy as its way to govern, which resulted in one of the greatest political advances in human history. All people are considered equal and deserve representation in political decision making. Accordingly, the system honors individuals and attempts to integrate their personal viewpoints into agreements that reflect the collective interests of the whole. In these ways, democracy reflects the processes of evolution that integrate separateness through relationships into more complex wholes.

During the last thirty years, the principles of democracy have been significantly eroded, as the democratic system has evolved to function increasingly like a plutocracy in which the wealthy significantly rule. The following ten-tier system provides examples of factors that have undermined our democracy in relation to citizens electing political representatives:

1. The politician with the most *money* typically wins the election. Therefore, money often determines elections before we even vote.

2. *Special interests* normally provide the money to the candidate. This arrangement means that the allegiance of the politician often falls primarily to the special interest, instead of to the voter. This allegiance likely continues as long as the politician seeks money as the lifeblood for future elections. Similarly, if the politician intends to seek future private employment affiliated with the special interest, the monetary allegiance continues even further.

3. The *Supreme Court ruling in Citizens United* in 2010 enabled corporations, labor unions, and wealthy individuals to donate unlimited funds to political organizations to either support or defeat a political candidate. These unlimited contributions often appear to be used to attack opposing candidates via negative advertising. The results of the special interest negative advertising often undermine constructive dialogue, honesty, cooperation, and trust necessary for an effective democracy. At the same time, it distracts voters from the crucial issues that need to be solved.

4. *Political parties* expect allegiance to their party politics in exchange for monetary and other support to the candidate, thereby further usurping the influence of the voting public.

5. *Fund-raising* can turn into a second job, as the politician prepares for future election campaigns. The time and energy expended on fund-raising interferes with the primary job of representing the interests of the voting public.

6. *Gerrymandering* election districts favor the election of particular political parties, thereby eroding the choices and influence of many voters while further obligating the candidate's allegiance to the party.

7. *Voter registration, identification requirements, and harassment* sometimes restrict eligible voters from participating in democratic processes.

8. *Vote counting* has developed into a significant issue, as demonstrated by the example of the Supreme Court deciding the 2000 presidential election.

9. The *Electoral College system* provides states rather than citizens the ultimate vote for President, thereby, diminishing the power of the vote for individual citizens.

10. *Voters* finally have their say in the election of the candidate. Unfortunately, the voting public—as the real constituents—may stand as deep as tenth in line to elect our "democratic" representative.

Conscious Evolution toward Democratic Rule

The time has come to return the political system to a democracy. Our health and sustainability depends upon this evolutionary step in which we invite all citizens to participate equally and take responsibility in the decision making processes of the nation. Democracy provides the opportunity for the natural competition for political power to evolve via cooperative voting procedures to elect representatives. These separate representatives then cooperate to make decisions for the whole. These collective decisions transcend and include the diversity of individual and special interests. Thus, democracy reflects the evolutionary processes in which separate individuals participate in cooperative relationships in efforts to contribute to the whole. In contrast, when competition persists and fails to advance into cooperation, the democratic system cannot consciously evolve and risks devolution.

Public Financing of Elections as an Important Step toward Democracy

To transition back toward the ideal of democratic rule requires that we control the influences of "Money and special interests" within the political system (see Figure 9). In addition, we can recreate our democracy by transferring power back to the people. An initial step proposed for this process involves the "Public financing" of elections. In other words, the public pays for elections and then votes to elect their representatives. In this way, politicians become dependent on and responsible to the public. Citizens pay for the elections and deserve to receive the benefits. This monetary role for the public invites more enthusiastic participation of citizens that introduces the potential to revitalize our democracy. The public financing of elections can be crafted in ways that prevent money, special interests, and political parties from substantially influencing the functioning of our democracy. Although challenges will no doubt arise relative to the public funding of elections, these problems will be minor in comparison to the present "democracy" that values money and special interests over our citizens, the world, and a healthy sustainable future.

In addition to initiating public funding of elections, we can similarly work to improve the first nine steps of the current election process. In these ways, we can consciously evolve our political system and revitalize our democracy, so it functions in integrity with the principle: of the people, by the people, and for the people.

Media

The media represent the primary sources of information about the world that exists beyond our personal experiences. As a consequence, the media have significant powers to shape our personal reality and in turn influence our behaviors regarding others, society, and the planet. Due to this extraordinary power to influence, the media possess the potential to move us toward continued evolution—or, in contrast, toward devolution.

Mission of the Media—Provide Full, Accurate Portrayals of Reality

Since conscious evolution depends upon increases in our awareness of *reality*, the media need to follow the lead of evolution and provide information that helps us understand the world more fully and accurately. In this way, the media have a natural higher purpose to provide information that facilitates human and evolutionary growth. To accomplish this mission, the media need to collect and share the most accurate, comprehensive information available. This information includes how special interests connect with collective interests to form the interests of the whole.

A more specific example of this evolutionary process involves the media telling a story of how a creative idea or innovation competes with other possibilities until cooperation accelerates its organization, order, and eventual oneness to transform into operating congruently in a more complex whole. In such ways, the media can help people understand and choose how to integrate their separateness through relationships into higher functioning wholes that promote living in harmony with others and the world.

In contrast, when the media frequently present separate special interest views of *reality*, these partial truths often intensify our perceptions of separateness. Such perspectives that highlight selective, limited viewpoints invite conflicts and competition with other special interest viewpoints. The win-lose conflicts that result can stall in the competition phase and fail to develop the necessary cooperation for successful evolution to proceed. Instead of evolution, the conflicts increase the risks of devolution. For instance, when conflicting parties perceive and act on limited versions of separateness, the risks increase that damages will occur to people and the environment.

The media possess profound responsibilities. They provide information about the world and *reality*, commonly not directly available to the public. The information provided often influences the evolution of the consciousness and actions of individuals, groups, cultures, and the global community. Consequently, the media need to honor a value system in which they present the "truth" in the most full, accurate forms possible, so they promote healthy sustainable living that increases our coherence with *reality*.

Four Competing Value Systems Undermine this Important Mission of the Media

In contrast to this ideal value of the media reporting as fully and accurately as possible regarding *reality*, four competing value systems have developed that severely compromise this principle. The capitalist system significantly influences each of these competing value systems. Consequently, these four competing values inadvertently introduce increased risks for devolution while they undermine the larger mission of the media.

1. The first competing value system involves *money*. Similar to the democratic institution in which money competes and undermines the goal for governance by and for the people, the media also normally rely on money for their lifeblood. This dependence on money can compromise the larger mission. For instance, media producers typically have to make money in order to survive in our capitalist system. This means that the survival, maintenance, and growth of the institution sometimes conflicts with the value to provide full, accurate information to the public. When the life of the media institution (actually an artificial life created by humans) seems threatened due to the lack of money or profits, efforts to save the institution can take priority over the ultimate mission of

the institution. In other cases, the growth and even the maintenance of the institution sometimes take precedence over providing high-quality information to the public.

2. In the United States, six *corporations* now control ninety percent of the media (Daly, Martenson, Fitz-Gerald, and Moors, 2012). This means that a miniscule number of special interest companies, with unknown agendas and filters on how they decide to define the "truth" of *reality*, disseminate information to the public. With new knowledge doubling approximately every eighteen months (Wilson, 2009), how well do they keep us informed of these enormous changes in the knowledge base regarding *reality* and the changing world?

3. The money that serves as the lifeblood of the media institution derives significantly from external *special interest groups*. For example, other special interest corporations and individuals desiring to market and sell products and services often advertise through the media. To protect this stream of advertising income, the media have to be cautious not to offend the advertisers with the information they present to the public. As a result, the flow of complete and accurate information can be compromised.

   Advertisers frequently utilize marketing techniques that appeal largely to base emotions and the sensate, bodily concerns of consumers. Examples of these marketing styles include a focus on food (e.g., survival and pleasure), sex appeal (e.g., love, pleasure, and survival), immediate gratification (e.g., pleasure and avoidance of pain), conflict arousal (e.g., fear and conquest), seeking status and wealth (e.g., worth and power), and success and winning (e.g., power and worth). These appeals stimulate our emotional and sensate brain functions to dominate our attention.

   Meanwhile, our creative, thinking, and integrative brain functions remain largely neglected. Unfortunately, these latter functions represent the primary sources of creativity, cooperation, and organizing abilities necessary for successful evolutionary growth. In contrast to the information that appeals to these more advanced evolutionary brain functions, information directed to the emotional and sensate functions tend to arouse feelings designed to stimulate the consumer to make a purchase. Nevertheless, the emotional and sensate functions have limited abilities to perceive *reality* fully enough to consider any long-term consequences of the purchase. Such emotionally driven consumption often increases the risks for devolutionary outcomes.

4. *Consumers* represent the fourth level of competition that often undermines the media from presenting the "truth" in more complete and accurate forms. In this case, consumers have a human brain that evolutionarily functions with emotions and bodily sensations as more deeply rooted, or defaulted, than the more advanced thinking, creative processes. Therefore, advertising that appeals to the emotional and sensate functions tend to stimulate consumers to attend to that message. The complex thinking and planning processes essential to guide us into a sustainable future recede into the background, as the emotional, sensate functions react to the advertising.

   In addition, as described earlier in reference to dependence and addiction tendencies, habits can form in relation to both material and information consumption. When information on the emotional, sensate levels stimulates the consumer to purchase the product, immediate gratification often occurs. Typically, the satisfaction soon dissipates, and the urge to consume arises again. A cycle of consumption may develop, as separate individuals naturally desire relationship connections that lead to a sense of oneness or fullness. These desires and their fulfillment through consumption can temporarily produce a sense of satisfaction. Nonetheless, the deeper sense of emptiness and isolation normally present in separate individuals can return and reinitiate the cycle of desire-consumption-satisfaction-emptiness. A dependent or addictive habit may begin to develop that offers temporary relief, and even pleasure, relative to the normal state of separateness.

When a cycle of consumption occurs in relation to the emotional and sensate brain functions, this cycle often contrasts with habits formed relative to the thinking, creative, and integrating functions. For instance, the emotional and sensate functions enjoy the experience, but the stimulation usually quickly fades. As a result, a cycle of consumption can arise that depends on the purchase or use of the external product again.

In contrast, the creative, thinking, and integrating functions have the capacity to hold onto the product or service neurologically in a way that the information can then be built upon internally through creative associations and personal growth. This means the cycle of dependency can shift from dependence on external materials to dependence on information internal to the person. With the information remembered by our brain, we can simply access it anytime we choose. We no longer have to purchase more goods and services. We can avoid dependence on external material resources that invite higher risks for devolution, especially when they involve finite, material resources.

As a result, our more complex cognitive functions can benefit, as they recall the stored information and creatively build upon it. For instance, we can experience pleasure from reading a stimulating novel or engaging with a compelling theory, as alternative forms of satisfaction compared to purchasing a sandwich or a sports car (Bougsty-Marshall, 2012). We can then communicate with others regarding the novel or the theory and generate further ideas that promote our personal and collective growth. Such internal growth in our consciousness can help us cocreate and evolve the world toward a healthy sustainable future.

Codependent Relationships among the Media, Advertisers, and Consumers

These four competing value systems—money, corporate ownership of the media, special interests, and consumers—undermine the larger mission of the media to share accurate, comprehensive information with the public. Instead, money drives each of the actors to take care of their special interests as a priority. Advertisers attempt to sell more products and services to consumers for more profits. This encourages both advertisers and the media in their mutual codependence to disseminate information that appeals significantly to the emotional, sensate brains of consumers. Since these brains are more easily influenced and offer increased opportunities to develop dependencies on the products and services, expanded profits can result. Hence, the media, advertisers, and consumers often work in mutually codependent relationships that serve the special interests of each party.

Unfortunately, this collection of special interests, although seemingly productive from an economic standpoint, unsuspectingly invites devolutionary consequences. Evolution depends largely on the creative, thinking, and integrating brain functions to initiate changes that culminate in sustainable growth. Since these brain functions often receive only selective and incomplete information from most of the media, they lack the full, accurate data necessary to evolve in healthy sustainable manners. If emotional, sensate advertising leads to addictive consumption, this development increasingly limits healthy, evolutionary growth. Simultaneously, it increases the risks for devolution.

Solutions That Support the Evolutionary Mission of the Media

Since our ultimate concern involves living a healthy sustainable life, the media can play a crucial role in pursuing this paramount goal. The media enjoy unique opportunities to inform us about the world beyond our personal experiences. Hence, accurate information that portrays the world as completely as possible depends upon a willing and competent media guided by this overriding mission. Only when we perceive *reality* accurately and fully can we act in integrity with what supports all our lives.

The media are often enmeshed in codependent relationships with advertisers and consumers, as each pursues money and their special interests. Nevertheless, the overarching goal to strive toward healthy sustainable living must be enacted from higher states of consciousness that focus on the collective interests of the public and the planet. The media need to recognize and take responsibility for their crucial role in the evolution or devolution of humanity. To support successful evolution the media must function consistent with evolutionary processes, ideally guided by the visionary purpose to create a healthy sustainable future. They also need to overcome the four competing systems—money, corporations, special interest groups, and consumers—that sometimes claim their special interests as more important than the collective interests, as well as more important than full, accurate versions of *reality*.

Unfortunately, the power of special interests and money may require a greater power to redirect them to serve the collective good. This greater power typically comes in the form of the government, whether local, state, national, or international. Nonetheless, special interests often protest and attempt to block any efforts to restrict their activities. The immediate crisis pertaining to the special interest concerns often seems to take precedence over the long-term harm to the collective, even though harm to the collective may eventually destroy the special interests.

Grassroots support will likely be necessary to encourage elected officials and special interests to act on behalf of the common good and the long-term sustainability of humanity. Elected officials and special interests exist due to the successful functioning of the collective society and planet. In other words, support for the collective actually supports the special interests and represents a prerequisite for their continued existence. Eventually, a general consensus can progressively develop in which collective interests are prioritized and healthy sustainable living becomes the paramount goal to guide the actions of all parties.

To encourage the media to follow this higher mission to deliver "Health & Sustainability news" (see Figure 9), the government can utilize a number of incentives. In general, laws can be developed, regulations enacted, and tax incentives provided to encourage media sources to act in service to the public. Grants and awards of recognition may help reinforce and motivate media institutions to educate effectively about *reality*.

Alternative media designed intentionally to provide more accurate, complete news coverage and documentaries to the public can be supported by private contributors, foundations, and grassroots movements. Meanwhile, the internet provides the greatest variety of possibilities to inform the public. Social media presents opportunities to democratize the media. Often free of monetary influences, the internet continually evolves with new information. It conveys not only more information from around the world, but has the potential to deliver and challenge people to evolve the information into higher levels of understanding.

For instance, increased quantities of separate information can be integrated into relationship and oneness perspectives. This integration of information to reflect *reality* more fully and accurately could substantially improve the efficiency and reliability of information shared. Such increased breadth and depth of understanding of the world can significantly enhance our capabilities to create a healthy sustainable future. With greater quantity and quality of information, we can learn to live in increased integrity with the whole that includes integrating our separateness, relationship interconnectedness, and our oneness into lifestyles that serve all people and the world.

Health Care

Health represents a fundamental, universal component of human life. It reflects how well we function overall and how well we operate in each of the twelve health dimensions that contribute to our lives (see chapter 4). These twelve dimensions include: physical, psychological, family, social, cultural, vocational, economical, political, recreational, environmental, spiritual, and ethical. They represent the basic ingredients that produce our overall health. Meanwhile, the functioning of the collection of these dimensions range along a health continuum from "life" at one end and "death" at the other end.

At the life end, ethical living promotes health for everyone and everything as we serve our fellow human beings and the planet as extensions of ourselves. In turn, ethical living benefits not only the receivers but the givers. When we give and improve the life of others and the environment, our health often benefits by experiencing greater meaning, satisfaction, and love. Reciprocally, the improved functioning of the recipients can then benefit our health. This ultimate form of health care integrates separateness, relationships, and oneness to create a unified process to help ourselves, others, the world, and evolution.

Next on the health continuum, optimal functioning maximizes our individual health (for example, through peak performance). Wellness involves the development of our personal capacities and skills so we experience productive, healthy living practices. Prevention efforts attempt to retain health in the presence of potential threats.

On the other hand, maintenance serves to stabilize our functioning into a comfort zone between growth and destruction. On the death end of the continuum, sickness entails several levels of functioning that range from distress to symptoms to disease to dying. Early intervention, treatment, rehabilitation, and hospice services intervene with these sickness conditions.

The Health Care System Developed into a Sickness Care System

Our present health care system functions primarily as a "Sickness care" system (see Figure 9). How is this possible, when people obviously function more effectively and productively on the positive life side of the health continuum? One explanation involves the historical development of health care. Originally, health care involved caring about the health of sick people and then taking actions to treat their maladies. Since sickness represents a natural part of life, treatment services have necessarily continued.

A second reason for the bias toward sickness care involves the influence of money. For instance, the exchange of money for medical treatment reinforced health care providers and eventually corporations to make a living treating sick people. No money was typically available, however, for prevention, wellness, optimal health, and ethical living interventions. Even if these interventions had been successfully provided, healthy people typically do not seek services. Hence, no customers for services results in no money. The economic livelihood of health care providers and corporations developed relative to the sickness side of the continuum, not the health side. As a consequence, the capitalist system has inadvertently reinforced services for sickness care but not for health promotion. The result is a "sickness care" institution.

Due to these influences, a pervasive sickness care system has developed and operates as a "health care system." Marvelous advances in treatment technologies, medications, and medical practices have developed. Meanwhile, the early successes of the medical treatment model cured broken bones and bacterial infections, as conditions with single causes. Unfortunately, treatment services usually fail to cure sicknesses that result from multiple causes, such as most chronic diseases. This means that despite the extraordinary efforts, technologies, and expenses utilized in the present health care system, symptom control instead of disease cures usually represent the norm.

With the underlying disease process continuing, the need to control symptoms soon becomes an ongoing process that perpetuates the need for treatments. So a dependency cycle often develops in which patients' desire ongoing treatment for symptom control, and ideally cures, while providers depend on the monetary profits from such treatment services to support their livelihoods. This treatment/profit cycle generates a mutual dependency between the patient and the health care providers. Much of the medical technology, pharmacological, insurance, and other support services of the health care system also operate within this dependency cycle. As a result, this cycle of treatment/profit dependency, combined with little or no profits associated with wellness interventions and healthy people, serve as fundamental drivers of our sickness care system.

This sickness care system naturally expands and, paradoxically, appears on a seemingly endless growth path. It largely fails to promote and keep people healthy. Furthermore, it often fails to help people avoid sicknesses and generally neglects to help people perform productively at their maximum capacities as workers and citizens. Instead, as people become sick, the system steps in to provide important treatment for their symptoms and suffering. Since the treatments usually do not address the multiple causes of most sicknesses and diseases, chronic treatment regimens can begin for chronic disease conditions. The treatment-profit system locks in place and leads to extraordinary costs both financially and in terms of suffering.

Economic Costs Associated with the Current Health Care System

The costs of the United States' health care system in 2009 came to $2.5 trillion, amounting to more than $8,000 per American and 17.6 percent of the gross domestic product (Centers for Medicare and Medicaid Services, 2009). "The United States spends significantly more on health care than any other nation … yet the average life expectancy in the United States is far below many other nations" (CDC, 2009b). Chronic diseases account for nearly three out of four deaths, as well as 75 percent of health care costs (CDC, 2007b). Five percent of the population spends nearly 50 percent of the health care dollars, while half the population spends nearly nothing (US

Department of Health and Human Services, 2007). "Four modifiable health risk behaviors—lack of physical activity, poor nutrition, tobacco use, and excessive alcohol consumption—are responsible for much of the illness, suffering, and early death related to chronic diseases" (CDC, 2012).

The Health Care System Appears Sick

Metaphorically, our overall health care system stands on the sickness side of the health continuum. The health side lacks the services to balance the over-weighted sickness side. Similar to an unbalanced teeter-totter, the entire system slowly slides toward the ground on the sickness side, where it faces possible bankruptcy. Consequently, the present health care system itself is "sick." It suffers from the distress naturally associated with sickness, as well as from negative symptoms such as the ever-expanding expenses associated with treatment services. Finally, it suffers from a disease process in which the chronic dependency of the treatment/profit cycle drives the institution toward financial and service delivery crises.

Sickness Care Evolves into Comprehensive Health Care

The health care system requires evolutionary reforms. We need to transform our current system from "sickness care" to a balanced system of "health care" (see Figure 9). This transformation depends upon the evolution of the health care system to embrace the entire health continuum. The foundation of a sustainable health care system depends on all the components along the health continuum functioning and balancing to maximize health outcomes. Accordingly, we need to evolve into a system in which we care about both health and sickness. This includes ethical living, optimal functioning, wellness, and prevention on the health end of the continuum, with maintenance as the fulcrum in the middle, and distress, symptoms, disease, and the death process on the sickness end.

Such a transformation in comprehensive health care could create a healthy and increasingly sustainable health care system. This evolved system naturally invests in human growth and health promotion, as well as in the prevention of sickness in order to create a balance between health and sickness care. Such a balance should not only improve the health of the population but transform the system into a genuine health care system.

As the health of people improves the need for expensive sickness care will likely diminish. Additionally, as health improves, productivity at work and effective functioning in other areas of life will likely follow. The overall health of the economy and the society will likely benefit, and in the process, these advances will promote further improvements in the health of citizens.

As improvements in individual and collective health occur, some special interest participants in the present health care system will likely suffer, unless they decide to evolve as well. The health care system will, thereby, expand care to include valuing positive health for people and the broader society, alongside continuing care for sick people.

The Health Continuum and Healthy Living Model Underlie Evolved Health Care

The kind of health care recommended here involves a balance of services across the health continuum. In addition, since healthy functioning depends on the twelve health dimensions, the healthy living model needs to be incorporated into the health care system. For instance, to improve the success of health care interventions across the health continuum, the twelve dimensions of the healthy living model provide a comprehensive tool for understanding how to best intervene to promote health and treat disease. The model can help assess what contributes to health at each component of the continuum. In this manner, the multiple contributing factors that lead to either health or sickness can be assessed and analyzed, so we can choose integrated interventions that cost-effectively improve functioning across the health continuum.

Ideally, this conception of health care can expand further to apply not only to individuals, but also to couples, families, groups, businesses, communities, nations, and even the entire world. Such a comprehensive, society-wide approach to the promotion of health can stimulate coordinated efforts to create synergies to improve health from the personal to societal to the global levels. Sickness care will continue, but will likely slow its rate of increases, as changing attitudes, behaviors, and lifestyles help improve the health of people. The promotion of health and the prevention of sickness, thereby, can help save lives, generate a productive workforce and society, as well as introduce more cost-effective and comprehensive service delivery.

Health Care That Aligns with Evolution Improves Health and Sustainability

From an evolutionary perspective (that extends beyond the priorities of our health, economic, and human viewpoints), we need to prioritize ethical living, optimal functioning, and wellness, as well as prevent sickness. Efforts to encourage positive growth correspond with the natural processes of evolution that progress into more unified, complex functioning. If we invest in the growth side of the health continuum, we encourage the cooperation and organization necessary to promote unified functioning at more complex levels. As we align more consistently with how evolution progresses, we naturally move toward increasing healthy sustainable living.

Health can also be examined more specifically in the context of the three dynamic processes of evolution—growth, maintenance, and destruction. For instance, destruction inherently occurs in the impermanence of evolutionary form, as death recycles present forms to serve as resources for future growth. The natural destruction process functions continuously and pulls us toward death. Therefore, if we simply attempt to maintain and survive in life, we maintain while unsuspectingly slipping toward our death. As a result, growth presents opportunities to evolve rather than devolve and offers our best hope to postpone death. Similarly, growth helps us minimize and avoid sickness that occurs along the path to death.

When we operate our health care system with the priority to treat sickness, we metaphorically engage in a fight with the evolutionary process of destruction that has already gained a foothold in winning the life-or-death battle. Sickness indicates that we have lost enough healthy functioning in aspects of our lives that destruction has pulled us along the path toward death. Unless we have come to terms with our death and intend to die with dignity, we naturally engage in the battle—the battle for our life. Nevertheless, at this point, the fight will likely prove expensive, arduous, and damaging, especially compared to our options to grow and maintain health. Only occasionally does the fight result in liberation in which we win, so we can prepare for future battles with sickness.

In contrast, when we invest in prevention, wellness, optimal functioning, and ethical living, we proactively counter the destruction process. With these choices, we step onto the natural path generated by evolution. We proceed along that route by increasing our consciousness, creativity, competition, cooperation, organization, order, and oneness (see figures 2 and 3). Through following these steps along the evolutionary path, we progress beyond our separateness (that is, our problem) and engage in relationships that can connect us into greater oneness with all that we perceive. In this process of growing from separateness to relationships to oneness, we cocreate and progress in the direction of healthy sustainable living. We can intentionally evolve our health care institution, as well as other societal institutions, to align with these natural growth steps that follow the lead of evolution. When we do so, we significantly expand our potential to create a successful future for all.

Education

Our education system serves as the primary institution for transferring information and knowledge systematically from one generation to the next. This transfer of personal and collective realities serves to promote human evolution, yet the information transmitted in most education institutions conveys narrow versions of *reality*. The normal information taught provides the basics of the three Rs ("reading, 'riting, and 'rithmetic"). Although these important thinking functions provide necessary tools for understanding and communicating about *reality*, they omit or neglect most of the other critical perceptual windows into the universe. Our evolutionary brain development provides the following windows into interpreting *reality*: sensory and kinesthetic; feelings and social; creativity and imaging, thinking and logic, witnessing and integrating; as well as meditative witnessing perspectives of *reality*.

Education Needs to Teach through All the Windows That Reveal Reality

If we continue to teach predominantly through one window into *reality*, we will fail to develop our capabilities to live in integrity with the world—we will instead invite devolution. We will also fail to realize our full potential as well as lack the capacities to integrate our brain functions to maximize healthy living. We must develop an education system that comprehensively teaches and integrates information through all our major windows that perceive *reality*. If we intend to be successful with the visionary goal to create healthy sustainable living, we need an education system that teaches how to understand and live in harmony with the entire world.

Traditional Education Primarily Prepares Students for Vocational Success

Historically, our education system evolved during the Industrial Age and helped prepare students to succeed in a capitalist economic system. In this context, rational thinking, communicating, and following the lead of an authoritarian or authoritative teacher provided important skills to help students succeed in the workplace. In the business world, a boss (teacher) usually gives directions to employees (students) who must follow orders or risk reprimand and eventually termination (poor grades and flunking out). In other words, our education system evolved significantly as a "Vocational training" system to help students prepare to be productive employees (see Figure 9).

Education Reform Supports the Vision for Healthy Sustainable Living

While the present education system supports the American Dream for success that prioritizes economic and vocational achievement, it is not sufficient to develop the universal vision for healthy sustainable living. The development of a healthy future depends upon effective functioning and balancing across all twelve universal dimensions of health. Since our present education system does not teach knowledge and skills that improve functioning in most of these health dimensions, the system will fail to bridge us into a healthy sustainable future.

As a consequence, we need our education system to evolve to teach how to develop and integrate our complex lives into healthy living. This means that we learn to manage our intellect in the interactive context of our emotional, social, financial, environmental, and physical lives. When we learn to live as a whole person, we create multiple opportunities to pursue happiness and fulfillment that can then benefit others and the world. In these ways, we progress far beyond the opportunities generally provided by our present education system and our workplace experiences.

The Education System Needs to Operate Consistently with Evolution

We need to evolve our education system and prioritize comprehensive "Healthy sustainable living training." This requires us to integrate the principles of healthy sustainable living into existing curriculums, as well as develop new curriculums. Such programs need designed for age-appropriate learning focused on selected issues within each of the twelve dimensions of health. For instance, preconception-to-cradle-to-grave curriculums, especially for young children and their parents, could provide critical learning opportunities at key developmental periods.

Teaching how the dimensions relate and how they complement or detract from each other can facilitate understanding the power of relationships. Learning how the health dimensions work together to form a whole that functions as more than the sum of its parts will provide a model to help comprehend how to live fully. The process of learning how separate dimensions cooperate in relationships to form a complex whole provides experiential examples of how evolution works. We can then perceive *reality* more fully and accurately, so we can choose actions consistent with positive evolutionary change.

Full-Brain Learning Promotes Progress toward Healthy Sustainable Living

In contrast to the teaching style associated with the three Rs that focuses primarily on the thinking function of the brain, full-brain learning needs to be promoted. We consider the learning capacity of each brain function to be important for developing our capabilities in that area, as well as for our overall functioning. For instance, as we develop our thinking capacities through normal education programs, we can intentionally support the development of our creativity and nonlinear brain functions by supporting our imagination and artistic expression. Similarly, we can develop the feeling functions and integrate the subjective world of emotions into the objective world of logical thinking. Teaching focused on our emotional intelligence can enlist our feelings to function as strengths to motivate learning rather than stimulating frequent distractions in the classroom. Our sensing and kinesthetic brain functions can help, again by avoiding distractions that manifest as behavior problems, and convert this energy into a window for experiential learning. Students can also learn to translate what the thinking brain learns and integrate this knowledge with the other brain functions.

We maximize our learning capacities when we utilize and then integrate our brain functions that interpret *reality*. When we perceive through our thinking, imaging, feeling, sensing, and integrating windows, we access unique views of the same material and information. When we integrate these different views of *reality* through a full-brain learning approach that synthesizes separate views and their relationships into greater oneness, we increase the fullness and accuracy of our picture of the "truth." In addition, we comprehend and retain the information more completely and with greater meaning. Furthermore, we can then increasingly understand how to solve problems and make more informed decisions regarding responsible uses of the information. We can consciously choose actions that increasingly harmonize with *reality*. Thus, we can use full-brain learning to increase our capabilities to recognize and avoid harm, as we contribute beneficially to ourselves, others, and the world.

From the practical standpoint, students tend to learn best based on their particular learning styles. For instance, some students learn most readily through kinesthetic touch and bodily actions. Others learn naturally through nonlinear, imaginative processes that contrasts with the linear logic usually taught in schools. As a result, teaching that adapts to and corresponds with the natural predispositions regarding how students learn, especially those who struggle to learn through their thinking function, could help students learn the 3 Rs more readily. Forcing students to learn through the traditional thinking function that appears as a less clear window to them produces less effective and efficient learning. Furthermore, the results often diminish their motivation to learn, undermine the development of their natural potentials, lower their self-esteem, and may even lead to dropping out of the education process.

A full-brain approach introduces students to learn more readily as they utilize their stronger learning capacities to access information based on their clearest windows into *reality*. The information can then be integrated across the different brain functions to ground it in the multiple perspectives provided by sensations, feelings, images, thoughts, and all their combinations. These multiple grounding points then provide various access sites to improve recall of the information. In addition, this approach generates numerous incubators for potential creativity as new associations among these different views can lead to innovative realizations. Such full-brain learning can generate new awareness and understandings of *reality* that motivate further learning, improved understanding, and greater development of living fully.

Developing our prefrontal lobes stands as crucially important, as they provide the capacities to witness, plan, solve problems, and integrate all the brain functions to work as a whole. They enable us to manage and direct the functions to serve higher purposes than immediate gratification of sensate, emotional, social, and fantasy desires. As students learn to manage their behaviors through prefrontal controls, teachers will be able to teach rather than engage in so much behavior management in the classroom. Both teaching and learning can improve. The prefrontal lobes also appear necessary to expand our consciousness to follow the natural path of evolution that integrates the three perspectives of separateness, relationships, and oneness. Breakthroughs in our conscious development in understanding and harmonizing with *reality*, therefore, depend substantially upon our prefrontal lobes.

Beyond the previous improvements recommended for brain functioning, the awareness provided by the functions of the mind enable us to witness energy and information of the world beyond the normal functioning of our sense organs. Accessing information directly from the world depends largely upon meditation and contemplation practices. These practices facilitate simple witnessing without attaching to and following the perceptions and interpretations of our normal brain functions—thinking, imaging, feeling, and sensations. When we do not attach to the information associated with our present brain functions, our awareness can sometimes access information that exists beyond what we normally perceive and already know. Opportunities to develop these inherent capacities, so we can access and more fully understand *reality* appear crucial for developing a sustainable future.

We also need to learn about our evolutionary brain and understand several devolutionary predispositions that threaten our future. For instance, we need to learn about how the amygdala, as an important memory organ, can automatically react to save our life from imagined death threats with fight, flight, and freeze reactions. Such strong, often inappropriate reactions can stimulate others to react in reciprocal manners, begetting vicious cycles that can lead to violence or, conversely, to the avoidance of solving problems. In a world in which we have created weapons, especially ones capable of mass destruction, we have a responsibility to learn how to retrain our brains to respond in appropriate manners that support a sustainable future.

Evolution Requires Schools to Evolve

Schools need to evolve and teach relevant information based on the twelve natural dimensions of our lives to engage and challenge students with real-world concerns. Learning about important life issues naturally invites students to increase their motivation for learning, as well as develop their proficiencies to create successful lives. Teaching them about *reality* as much as possible invites them to develop their consciousness and actions skills. They can then choose how to contribute to a healthy, productive, and peaceful world—for their own sake and for the sake of all humanity and evolution.

Furthermore, evolution predisposes growth as a natural function. Conscious evolution depends upon the expansion of our awareness. Our consciousness grows as we learn more about *reality* and increasingly perceive the whole. Such learning improves our abilities to understand and participate in the world in ways that promote evolution and not devolution.

Learning occurs best through full-brain functioning. As we integrate our thinking, imaging, feeling, and sensing functions, our brain evolves internally with neural networks (Hanson, 2012) to create increasingly full, accurate versions of *reality*. As we integrate these separate brain functions through interconnected relationships we develop an increasingly unified personal reality. In this way, our internal learning can correspond with the natural processes of evolution by integrating separate bits of information through relationships with other brain functions to form a more complex, unified picture of the issue. From this integrated conceptualization we can choose what actions to initiate in the external world in efforts to transform its separate parts into interactive relationships that contribute to the constructive functioning of the whole situation. In these ways, full-brain functioning enables us to contribute to and integrate both internal and external evolutionary processes.

Conscious Evolution Depends upon Expansions in Consciousness via Meditation

The combination of how little we know about *reality* and the continuing emergence of devolutionary problems indicate that we need to learn more than these improved education methods can likely deliver. Accordingly, mind-expansion techniques, such as the following example, need to accompany these full-brain learning and healthy living approaches.

Traditional education relies predominantly on knowledge gathered through human history. Although important, this collective knowledge from the past can provide objective information about *reality*, but this knowledge needs complemented with direct experiential information that we can apply in the present. Awareness of the present moment appears essential if we intend to apply past knowledge effectively in the present, so we can evaluate how to create a viable future. To live in harmony with *reality* we need awareness of the past, the present, and the potentials of the future to cocreate in integrity with the evolutionary processes.

Consequently, we need to teach meditation and contemplation techniques so students develop their innate capacities for awareness of information present in the moment that they normally fail to perceive. This information may pertain to sensory, emotional, creative, and logic concerns that go unrecognized while memorizing the answer for the next test. Additionally, the information may involve potential answers to questions, problems, planning possibilities, or the realization of a prior goal. The answer may seemingly come from nowhere, as we access information in the universe normally beyond our awareness. Similar to attractor field practices in which we connect with energy of the same frequency, we resonate with information and energy that seems magically to fulfill our emotional, cognitive desires, and especially, our higher purposes.

Since healthy sustainable living depends upon increasingly full, accurate perceptions of *reality*, we need to learn to access more information than we presently do through our sense organs. In the future, the most important "A" grade that we can achieve comes not from human teachers but from evolution and how we perform in relation to the world and *reality* as a whole.

Students and Teachers Need to Practice Healthy Sustainable Living

The healthy living dimensions can come alive in the school through the teachers and administrators actually practicing these principles. This living-the-teaching method could accelerate learning for students and staff alike. Along these lines, both teachers and students could complete the

Healthy Living Questionnaire to accelerate understanding how to develop healthy living (see Bougsty, 2012). The survey assesses individual functioning across the twelve health dimensions to identify existing strengths and weaknesses. Goals can then be set to reinforce as well as improve functioning among the different dimensions and their interactive balance necessary to realize healthy living. Actions steps can be specified and prioritized to develop a coordinated, synergistic approach to improve healthy functioning. The questionnaire can also be utilized on the organizational level to assess and plan how to improve the school's health and functioning for the staff, the students, the parents, and the community.

In these ways, students can learn and practice healthy living in their real-life relationships at school. Students can learn healthy practices in their physical, psychological, social, financial, and emerging vocational lives, as they also learn to care, empathize, cooperate, and problem solve in teamwork with others. This comprehensive, dynamic teaching environment can transcend academic knowledge and convert objective information into subjective and collective experiences, as students and teachers practice healthy living. In these ways, teaching can eventually be easier, more effective, and enriching for all concerned.

Teachers still need to share traditional reductionism science that presents objective findings to understand the parts of the whole. When appropriate, these teachings can be extended with social science, systems theory, and holistic and quantum science to understand the relationships and whole functioning involved. In addition, teachers need to develop the capabilities to shift from authoritative to democratic teaching styles that facilitate students learning experientially, integrating their brain functions, developing their creativity, and working collectively as teams to complete projects.

Furthermore, specialists may temporarily be required to teach meditation skills to help students access their natural capacities to experience the world beyond their sense organs and normal conceptualizations of *reality*. Meditation can accelerate our progression from egocentric to ethnocentric to worldcentric to kosmocentric stages of consciousness faster than any other method (Wilber, 2006). In these ways, students can start developing their intuitive, creative, visionary, and eventually, nondual capacities to perceive *reality* more fully and accurately to increase their conscious abilities to live in interdependent relationships with others and the world.

Specific teachings and practices on how to develop, maintain, as well as continue to grow into healthy sustainable living will be essential to prepare people to create conscious lifestyles. Healthy living will transcend and include the former career development performed by schools. Finally, schools represent the most universal institution to prepare and transform students, the parents, society, and the world to act responsibly and wisely in efforts to cocreate a healthy sustainable future.

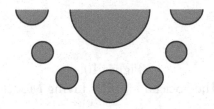

CHAPTER 8

The Societal and Comprehensive Healthy Living Models

• • • • • • •

Healthy Living on All Levels of Society

The healthy living model (see figure 5) identifies the twelve universal dimensions of health, including physical, psychological, family, social, cultural, vocational, economical, political, recreational, environmental, spiritual, and ethical. These dimensions need to function individually as well as synergize in mutually supportive relationships, and ultimately balance into a whole system of health.

The healthy living model applies initially to individuals. Nevertheless, since individuals generate activities on all levels of human society, the twelve dimensions of health apply to all. Thus, healthy living functions on each level of society, interrelates across levels, and culminates in healthy living for the society as a whole. Thus, healthy living can be assessed, planned, and monitored on each and every level of the society through the use of the Healthy Living Questionnaire (Bougsty, 2012). To improve our abilities to understand how these different levels of healthy living interrelate we can see the Societal Healthy Living Model (Figure 10).

The Societal Healthy Living Model

This integrated societal model demonstrates the same basic, evolutionary structure as the original model. In this case, the separate parts consist of the twelve dimensions of health that also operate within six separate levels of society. These levels include "Self," "Family," "Business," "Community," "Nation," and the "World." They function in interdependent relationships, within each level and between all the levels, as they affect the health of humanity as a whole. When the multidimensional parts and their interdependent relationships improve in their functioning, the health of the whole tends to improve. As overall health improves, efforts to maintain these gains can contribute to their sustainability. With the maintenance of these new creations, a stable foundation can form from which further growth and evolution can proceed.

Figure 10:
The Societal Healthy Living Model

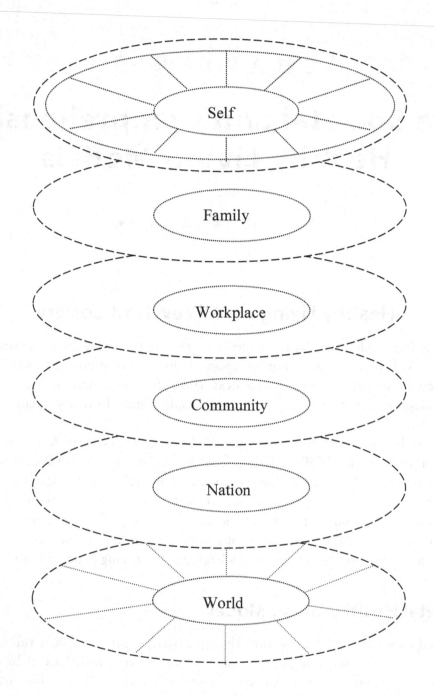

Healthy Sustainable Living Emerges from a Growth-Maintenance-Growth Cycle

This growth-maintenance-growth cycle parallels the natural growth processes of evolution. As creative changes maintain themselves, they stabilize as sustainable changes. Destruction processes tend to diminish their effects and a virtuous cycle can develop in which the separate parts, their relationships, and the whole can evolve progressively into higher functioning. When these changes maintain and function as a more orderly whole, then the whole becomes a ground for future growth. Through such growth-maintenance-growth cycles, healthy sustainable living progressively manifests.

The evolution of individual and societal health can follow these same basic processes. For instance, from the perspective of individual health, enhanced functioning within the twelve dimensions, as well as synergistic growth among the dimensions, can improve the overall health of the individual. From the perspective of society, health also progresses when we improve functioning at more inclusive levels of humanity. For example, if we improve the health of the family, we likely also increase the health of the family members. More broadly, when we improve healthy functioning at the community level, we often enhance the health of multiple families, as well as their members, simultaneously.

The Worldcentric Stage of Consciousness Is Crucial for Creating a Viable Future

The stages of consciousness from which we normally perceive the world also affect our ability to grow and evolve. For instance, the worldcentric perspective creates the opportunity to perceive and value all people and the planet. In contrast, the ethnocentric and egocentric perspectives typically perceive the special interests of groups or individuals, respectively. The worldcentric perspective, portrayed by the societal healthy living model, introduces a comprehensive overview of human activities from which to evolve our health. This model enables us to contemplate different dimensions and different levels of the world community, so we create the opportunity to integrate our actions into *reality* more harmoniously and, in the process, generate increasingly healthy sustainable outcomes.

To succeed as a species, we must expand our perceptions to the worldcentric level in which we consider the health and needs of all people (Wilber, 2006). Such global efforts to create health and sustainability represent an essential investment in our future. Therefore, the traditional, narrow focus on individual health, although still necessary and important, gives way to more comprehensive understandings of healthy living across the world community. Only when we perceive *reality* as fully and accurately as possible can we expect to maximize our potential to create a healthy sustainable future.

The Comprehensive Healthy Living Model

The societal healthy living model can further expand into the Comprehensive Healthy Living Model (Figure 11). This comprehensive model introduces a systematic means to select constructive actions across all the health dimensions and levels of society. Therefore, it provides a practical tool to help guide our conscious evolution efforts. The model appears as a three-dimensional cube. The twelve "Health Dimensions" and six "Levels of Society" represent two of the three sides of the cube. (Other levels of society, such as neighborhoods, organizations, and states, can be added or substituted for the six major levels, as appropriate to the situation of interest.) The combination of these health dimensions and different levels of society provide important assessment and planning tools to improve health from the local to the global levels. The third side of the cube exhibits three "Types of Interventions": "Wellness," "Prevention," and "Treatment." These choices improve our ability to meet the particular health needs on each level and across all levels of society.

Through this comprehensive model of health, we can systematically choose how to transform society towards healthy functioning. We can intervene in proactive, coordinated manners that simultaneously consider healthy living across the twelve dimensions, all levels of society, and across the health continuum from wellness to prevention to treatment options. In addition, this comprehensive portrayal of the major dimensions and levels of society facilitates us to perceive *reality*, without omitting crucial areas. From this increasingly full, accurate perspective, we can select actions more appropriately in efforts to realize our vision for the future of humanity.

The Comprehensive Healthy Living Model Provides Assessment, Planning, and Intervention Tools

This comprehensive model introduces the following opportunities for improving healthy living throughout society and the world:

- **Assessment tools** evaluate how these twelve dimensions operate and interact across the different levels of society that, in turn, facilitates us to:

  - Identify the causal factors that underlie problems that may threaten *destruction* and devolutionary consequences;

  - Assess what contributes to the *maintenance and sustainability* of our progress, as well as the preservation of our present living conditions; and

  - Select factors that can generate further *growth* that propel us toward healthy sustainable living.

- **Planning choices** analyze the strengths and weaknesses of different dimensions across various levels of society, so we can grow, maintain, and avoid destruction, as we pursue healthy sustainable living; and

Figure 11:
The Comprehensive Healthy Living Model

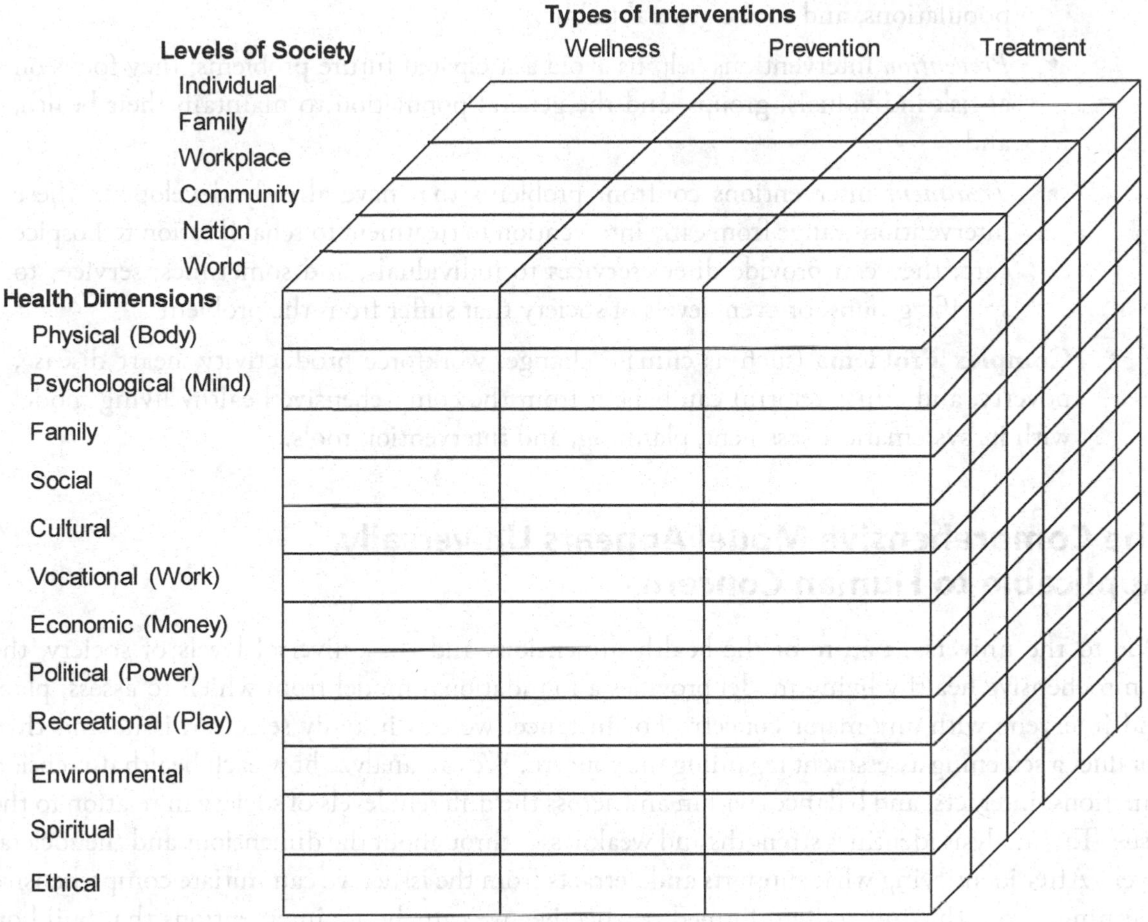

- **Intervention methods** introduce comprehensive choices about improving healthy living:
  - *Wellness* interventions promote healthy living. These interventions can encourage wellness, optimal functioning, and ethical living, and apply to individuals, specific populations, and to the general public.
  - *Prevention* interventions help us avoid anticipated future problems; they focus on at-risk individuals, groups, and the general population to maintain their health; and
  - *Treatment* interventions confront problems that have already developed. These interventions range from early intervention to treatment to rehabilitation to hospice care; they can provide direct services to individuals, and sometimes, services to specific groups, or even, levels of society that suffer from the problem.
- **Complex Problems** (such as climate change, workforce productivity, heart disease, poverty, and ethics reform) can benefit from the comprehensive healthy living model with its systematic assessment, planning, and intervention tools.

The Comprehensive Model Appears Universally Applicable to Human Concerns

Due to the universal nature of the health dimensions and the universal levels of society, the comprehensive healthy living model provides a foundational model from which to assess, plan, and intervene with any major concern. For instance, we can initially select an issue and then conduct a screening assessment regarding the concern. We can analyze how each health dimension functions, interacts, and balances within and across the different levels of society in relation to the issue. This analysis identifies strengths and weaknesses throughout the dimensions and the societal levels. After identifying what supports and detracts from the issue, we can initiate comprehensive planning. From this integrally informed perspective, we can choose interventions that build on the strengths, maintain successful gains, and treat important deficiencies. In these ways, we can systematically and comprehensively improve the functioning of whatever concern we choose. Since the model inherently values health across all levels of humanity, it supports our conscious evolution into an increasingly healthy future.

All Levels of the Society Affect Individual Health

All levels of society and the twelve dimensions interact and affect the health of the individual. For example, consider the health effects on the individual person from these multiple levels and dimensions of influence. Initially, the family usually serves as the first line of learning about health. If the family lacks healthy psychological and social skills, the individual will likely suffer deficiencies in these dimensions. If peers at school or work then perform in dysfunctional manners psychologically and socially, unhealthy beliefs and behaviors may solidify into increasingly chronic problems. If the community does not identify these problems and offer services to help the individual gain healthy psychological and social skills, then the individual will probably suffer diminished productivity as a citizen. Eventually, the individual may undermine health at various levels of society, as the person experiences a health care crisis, a divorce, or a workplace conflict.

In these ways, societal health affects individual health that, in turn, can affect the health of the society. Consequently, if we seriously want to improve our personal health, we need to assess and improve the functioning and balance of the twelve dimensions in our personal life, as well as improve healthy functioning throughout all levels of society that also affect our health.

Benefits Tend to Increase with Interventions at More Inclusive Levels of Society

In general, we gain the greatest health benefits when we prioritize planning and interventions at the highest level of society possible. For instance, when the nation's health suffers, the health of states, communities, businesses, all the way to the individual citizen will likely also suffer to some degree. Conversely, if the health of an individual suffers, the health of all the more complex, organized levels of society will likely suffer, yet, usually to a much lesser extent. Hence, each increase in complexity and inclusiveness of the level of society (for instance, the community level is more inclusive than the family, which is more inclusive than the individual) generally results in greater contributions to overall societal health. For example, if we intend to have the greatest influence to improve health in the society, then we need to plan and choose interventions initially at the national level (ideally, global level interventions can eventually be included).

As an example of how to improve healthy living throughout the nation, I will provide a collection of multi-level and multi-dimensional recommendations by using the Comprehensive Healthy Living Model. In the following section, I will introduce a combination of wellness, prevention, and treatment interventions in efforts to help guide the nation toward improvements in healthy living. These gains can accelerate by developing complementary recommendations for interventions across all levels of the society, including state, community, business, organization, family, and individual levels that can contribute to synergistic improvements in healthy living.

After the example of promoting healthy living on a national basis, I will provide a second example that demonstrates how to solve a specific societal problem. In this case, recommendations will be summarized on how to decrease the use of tobacco, as the most preventable form of death in the United States. The model can be employed in similar manners to enhance health on any particular level of society (like the community level), or within any dimension of health (for example, the psychological dimension), or pertaining to any special interest (such as health care reform or environmental impact assessments). Improved functioning on all levels of society and with all problems are necessary in order to move systematically toward the development of healthy sustainable living for all.

Comprehensive Healthy Living Applied to the Nation

The comprehensive healthy living model serves as a planning tool to help improve healthy functioning, in this case, improve healthy living throughout the nation. This example highlights the importance of addressing and integrating wellness, prevention, and treatment interventions. Such a comprehensive approach intentionally works to meet the diverse needs of the population, while not omitting any significant contributors to healthy living.

We normally rely on specialized approaches to improve functioning in our society. Unfortunately, inherent in specialization, interventions usually target only specific areas (for example, certain health dimensions and only select levels of society) and ignore other areas that also contribute to the problem. As expected, limited success normally results.

In contrast, this comprehensive approach introduces opportunities to produce significantly greater success. For instance, it includes and can address all twelve health dimensions and six major levels of society. Identifying contributions to the problem from each of these dimensions and levels can clarify specific interventions needed to solve the issue. In addition, this comprehensive approach also introduces a range of intervention possibilities for confronting the problem more precisely and systematically. In this case, wellness interventions serve to generate health and skill development, while prevention activities attempt to maintain our existing functioning whenever we anticipate difficulties. Finally, treatment interventions confront not only symptoms, but more importantly, root causes of the problem.

To keep this example simple, I will apply recommendations to the national level only. This means that the world level will be temporarily omitted, as seen in the abridged model presented in Figure 12. The community, business, family, and individual levels can accelerate the gains toward healthy living when recommendations on each of these levels coordinate with the national recommendations. Furthermore, interventions on additional levels that seem relevant, such as the regional, state, organizational, and neighborhood levels, can complement and extend the positive benefits generated by the national interventions.

The best results can be expected when recommendations from all the relevant levels integrate and synchronize. This means that comprehensive planning for wellness, prevention, and treatment interventions need developed for all the significant dimensions of health and levels of society in order to coordinate and synergize the interventions to produce maximal results. This integrated approach helps promote the success, as well as maximizes progress toward the development of healthy living throughout the nation.

Recommended Wellness, Prevention, and Treatment Interventions

Physical Dimension: The most important recommendation involves establishing "Healthy Sustainable Living (HSL)" as the overarching goal for the nation to pursue. This visionary goal (introduced as a wellness goal in the physical dimension of Figure 12) serves like a compass to orient and integrate all the interventions to work together to improve healthy functioning throughout the nation. Since well-intended interventions can also generate dangerous outcomes, we need the ethical living model (see chapter 9) to evaluate the potential for hidden, harmful consequences.

Meanwhile, "Health care reform based on Healthy Living (HL)" provides a prevention intervention associated with the physical dimension. When we ground health care reform in all the dimensions of life that contribute to physical health, we include yet transcend the medical model of health. Instead of focusing almost exclusively on the physical dimension and, in particular, on sickness, we gain the perspective of how different areas of life influence physical health. More importantly, we realize that all areas of life contribute to the health of the person as a whole. Furthermore, when we base health care reform on the principles of healthy living, we implicitly support movement toward healthy sustainable living.

Figure 12:
The Comprehensive Healthy Living Model: National Recommendations

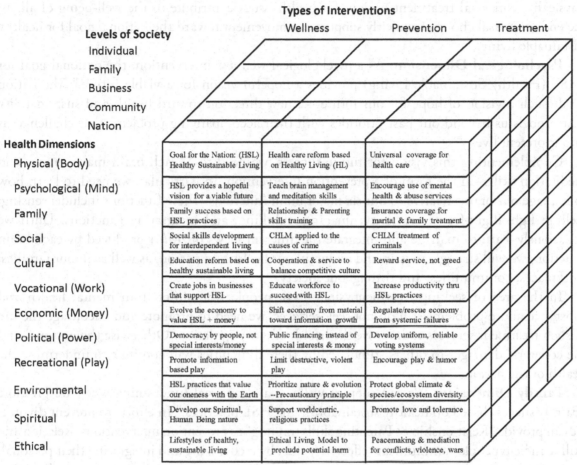

Types of Interventions

Levels of Society
Individual
Family
Business
Community
Nation

Health Dimensions

Health Dimensions	Wellness	Prevention	Treatment
Physical (Body)	Goal for the Nation: (HSL) Healthy Sustainable Living	Health care reform based on Healthy Living (HL)	Universal coverage for health care
Psychological (Mind)	HSL provides a hopeful vision for a viable future	Teach brain management and meditation skills	Encourage use of mental health & abuse services
Family	Family success based on HSL practices	Relationship & Parenting skills training	Insurance coverage for marital & family treatment
Social	Social skills development for interdependent living	CHLM applied to the causes of crime	CHLM treatment of criminals
Cultural	Education reform based on healthy sustainable living	Cooperation & service to balance competitive culture	Reward service, not greed
Vocational (Work)	Create jobs in businesses that support HSL	Educate workforce to succeed with HSL	Increase productivity thru HSL practices
Economic (Money)	Evolve the economy to value HSL + money	Shift economy from material toward information growth	Regulate/rescue economy from systemic failures
Political (Power)	Democracy by people, not special interests/money	Public financing instead of special interests & money	Develop uniform, reliable voting systems
Recreational (Play)	Promote information based play	Limit destructive, violent play	Encourage play & humor
Environmental	HSL practices that value our oneness with the Earth	Prioritize nature & evolution --Precautionary principle	Protect global climate & species/ecosystem diversity
Spiritual	Develop our Spiritual, Human Being nature	Support worldcentric, religious practices	Promote love and tolerance
Ethical	Lifestyles of healthy, sustainable living	Ethical Living Model to preclude potential harm	Peacemaking & mediation for conflicts, violence, wars

Treatment interventions in the physical health dimension can provide "Universal coverage for health care." We need to care for the health of all people, for moral and ethical reasons, but also because we live together, interdependently as a whole society. The health of each person, directly or indirectly, affects the health of others—economically, vocationally, socially, and physically. Universal treatment options for health issues contribute to the well-being of all. In the end, universal choices implicitly support our movement toward the national goal for healthy sustainable living.

Psychological Dimension: As a psychological wellness intervention, the national goal for "HSL (Healthy Sustainable Living) provides a hopeful vision for a viable future." The nation needs such a vision of hope for our future—a new direction toward health and sustainability that propels us beyond our past priorities with their accompanying problems that challenge us in our present lives.

Complementing this vision for future success, we need to "Teach brain management and meditation skills" in the form of a prevention intervention. In particular, we need to learn how to manage our brains relative to our six major brain functions. These functions include: sensing; feeling; fight-flight-freeze reactivity; imaging; thinking; and integrating functions. Until we consciously learn to manage and integrate the different views of *reality* produced by each brain function, we will struggle to gain and maintain our health as a person, as well as in our families, workplaces, communities, and throughout society.

In the area of seeking treatment, since most people who suffer from mental health and substance abuse problems still do not seek services, we need to promote and encourage the use of such treatment services to improve the health of our population. Otherwise the personal and the collateral damages to others stimulated by these difficulties will continue to undermine the health of the nation.

Family Dimension: We can support wellness and optimal functioning when we promote "Family success based on healthy sustainable living HSL practices." In efforts to prevent divorce, we can provide "Relationship & Parenting skills training" as prevention interventions. Relationship skills can help people communicate effectively (first by recognizing and integrating their personal, six brain functions) and then communicate as couples to create win-win outcomes. Training for parenting skills can then help children develop and integrate their brain functions, so they can manage their brains effectively and in healthy manners. Parents can learn how to help children through crucial development periods in their brain development and model healthy living, so the children naturally learn consistent with their stage of development. In these ways, children can grow into healthy, productive citizens who contribute to the creation of a healthy sustainable future. Treatment options that facilitate resolving family difficulties can be supported by "Insurance coverage for marital and family treatment."

Social Dimension: We can support wellness by providing "Social skills development for interdependent living." This means that we supply people with tools to help them negotiate how to live constructively with others and develop healthy win-win relationships. People can move beyond common codependent relationships and, instead, learn to embrace healthy, interdependent relationships. Such interdependent relationships grow out of independent people mutually choosing outcomes in which all win—the self, the other person, humanity, the planet, and evolution. Such win-win-win-win-win relationships promote our alignment with healthy sustainable living.

In the area of prevention, a practical use of the "CHLM (Comprehensive Healthy Living Model) applied to the causes of crime" helps identify the multiple underlying contributors to criminal activities. With comprehensive interventions we can start to prevent, rather than simply react, to these costly social problems. In addition, the comprehensive healthy living model used in the "CHLM treatment of criminals" can introduce a comprehensive means to assess, plan, and intervene to rehabilitate incarcerated people into more productive, healthy lifestyles.

Cultural Dimension: Wellness in the cultural dimension can support societal change through "Education reform based on healthy sustainable living." Such education can prepare citizens with the necessary tools to help themselves and society progress toward healthy sustainable lifestyles, responsible citizenship, and successful living. Part of this transformation process can involve a prevention shift toward "Cooperation & service to balance competitive culture," thereby balancing public interests with personal and special interests. In addition, we can make a treatment, cultural transition in which we increasingly "Reward service, not greed." We can begin to modify our tendencies toward greed and self-centered behavior and change into supporting other people and the environment. Since our lives ultimately depend upon others and the environment, such service represents an investment in us, as well as in the nation and the world.

Vocational Dimension: In the vocational dimension, a Wellness intervention involves the goal to "Create jobs in businesses that support HSL." In other words, we can develop a society in which the business sector overtly and substantively supports the long-term health and viability of the entire nation and the world. This means that we protect other people and the environment, as we produce goods and services.

To complement this goal, we can initiate a prevention intervention in which we specifically "Educate (the) workforce to succeed with HSL." In the end, businesses only succeed, if people and the environment succeed. This means that employers and employees must work together and prioritize the development of a healthy sustainable future. We can also teach businesses to "Increase productivity thru HSL practices" via treatment interventions that improve the functioning of employees, increase the satisfaction of customers, while promoting the protection of the environment. In these ways, businesses will succeed in the future by practicing win-win-win-win-win productivity and service delivery.

Economic Dimension: Wellness in the economic arena recommends that we "Evolve the economy to value HSL + money." Thus, healthy sustainable living ultimately becomes the driving force in the economy and money and profits function to serve this larger goal (see chapter 6).

A prevention intervention that promotes a sustainable economy means that we "Shift (the) economy from material toward information growth." Since material consumption depends upon finite material resources, limited supplies can fail to meet growing demands. A sustainable future, therefore, can be threatened if the economy continues to rely primarily on material growth, as shortages in products can sometimes stimulate environmental, political, and military conflicts. Instead, an economy based increasingly on information growth depends on what appears as infinite resources, as the potentials of our consciousness seem unlimited. Therefore, an economy that favors growth in information consumption, rather than material consumption, offers hope for a sustainable future.

In efforts to preserve the economy, a treatment option to "Regulate/rescue (the) economy from systemic failures" seems in order to protect the economic sustainability of national and international interests. In this context, appropriate regulations appear far favorable to a rescue mission during a crisis. The complex, interdependent nature of the economy upon which humanity has become dependent lacks healthy options to manage the destruction of a financial meltdown.

Political Dimension: In the political health arena, a wellness intervention involves the creation of a "Democracy by people, not by special interests/money." This means that people, rather than the influence of special interests and their money, run the country. Public interests of the majority, rather than special interests of the minority, then take priority. Nevertheless, since money presently serves as the lifeblood of elected officials in the United States, their allegiance to the power of special interest money substantially determines their political fate.

As a prevention intervention designed to ameliorate this flaw in our current political system, "Public financing instead of special interests & money" will help political leaders shift their focus from special interests to serve public interests, since the public will pay for their election campaigns (see chapter 7). Politicians will succeed based increasingly on their support for public interests, including healthy sustainable living goals, rather than support for special interest power and monetary contributions. In the treatment arena, we can also strengthen our democracy, if we "Develop uniform, reliable voting systems," including voter registration procedures.

Recreational Dimension: We can "Promote information based play" that expands the infinite reaches of our consciousness; this represents a wellness intervention in the recreational dimension. Such growth of our higher brain capacities supports the consciousness necessary to continue to expand toward healthy sustainable living. Such a priority in relation to information also supports the shift necessary in our economy to grow based increasingly on information rather than material consumption.

As a prevention option, we can "Limit destructive, violent play" that naturally develops our brain with neural networks related to violence and destruction. Instead, we can develop our nervous system to promote creative, cooperative problem solving that corresponds with contributing to a peaceful, sustainable world. As a treatment alternative, when people experience deficits in the recreational area, we can "Encourage play and humor" as a healthy antidote that may also include physical exercise to help counter obesity and various chronic diseases.

Environmental Dimension: "HSL practices that value our oneness with the Earth" represent wellness interventions in the environmental area. Such practices benefit the environment when we appreciate and act consistent with our natural interdependence with the planet. From our interconnected oneness, we behave as if the earth is an extension of ourselves and, reciprocally, that we are an extension of the earth. We protect the planet to protect ourselves.

Prevention efforts can "Prioritize nature & evolution—Precautionary principle" as fundamental to our lives. Physical and biological evolution has been tested successfully over millions and billions of years; meanwhile, cultural evolution has been tested for centuries, and recent technological innovations have been experimented with for years at the most. For instance, we have approved eighty-five thousand new synthetic chemicals with fewer than ten percent having been tested for their effects on human health. We have assumed innocence until proven guilty instead of assuming these mutations will perform like most mutations and fail, sometimes causing damage before they succumb to destruction. Consequently, we need to follow the "precautionary principle" that prescribes that we prevent and minimize harm rather than trying to manage damages after they occur (Commonweal, 2012).

In the treatment arena, we must "Protect global climate & species/ecosystem diversity," as these physical and biological systems influence our long-term sustainability. Presently, the loss of species in the world appears to occur at more than one thousand times the normal rate, and these extinctions result mostly from human activities. An estimated one in four mammals may "face a high risk of extinction in the near future" (The International Union for Conservation of Nature, 2012). Unfortunately, humans stand at risk in this mass-extinction process.

Fortunately, we have the opportunity to evolve consciously and choose healthy sustainable living, instead of our historic special interest, profit-and-consumption approach to living. Our special interest orientation has generated incredible success with cultural progress, yet inadvertently has stimulated most of these destructive outcomes. The ethical living model in chapter 9 and the integrated, healthy sustainable living model in chapter 10 introduce conscious evolution tools to help us predict and avoid these potentially deadly side effects.

Spiritual Dimension: In the spiritual realm, wellness interventions challenge us to "Develop our Spiritual, Human Being nature." This means that we develop and integrate our "doing" and "being" natures. For instance, our doing nature consists of any physical and mental activities in which we engage within our everyday evolutionary lives. Meanwhile, our being nature involves our simple awareness without attaching conceptualizations or actions. Such consciousness involves simple witnessing as practiced in many forms of meditation (Wilber, 2004). While being aware, we sometimes expand our consciousness in which we access more information from *reality* than we normally perceive. Thereby, we expand our repertoire of choices for what doing activities to initiate. Since we perceive more of *reality* than normal, we increase our opportunities to align with the world in more healthy sustainable ways. At the same time we increase our capacities to integrate our human and spiritual natures to enliven as a spiritual, human being.

Meanwhile, prevention in the spiritual domain recommends that we "Support worldcentric, religious practices." Since each major religion has developed worldcentric practices, followers need to care for their religious group and beliefs, as they also learn to care for other people and the whole world (Wilber, 2006). In this way, practitioners can take responsibility to steward all humanity and Earth "as God's creations." If practices that value the whole world fail to develop, then special interest orientations will prevail and perpetuate our current perceptions of separateness. Such special interest, separate perspectives neglect to perceive and value the interconnected, interdependent relationships and the functioning of the whole that keep us alive. Without perceiving and taking responsibility for our entire inherent nature—separateness, relationships, and oneness—we will continue to damage and destroy the life-support systems upon which our lives depend. Unbeknownst to us, we will likely be choosing extinction, instead of awakening to our opportunity to cocreate in conscious manners that benefit "all of God's creation."

Finally, to facilitate the advancement of spiritual practices throughout the world, a treatment approach invites us to "Promote love and tolerance" for other religions, as well as for all people and all participants in this evolutionary journey.

Ethical Dimension: Finally, the most important wellness intervention on the ethical dimension challenges us to develop and practice "Lifestyles of healthy sustainable living." Prevention efforts involve using the "Ethical Living Model to preclude potential harm" on all levels of society and all levels of evolution (examples can be found in chapters 9 and 10).

In conclusion, a treatment alternative for ethical living involves "Peacemaking & mediation for conflicts, violence, (and) wars." Peacemaking begins internally with the six major functions of our brain. These functions need to reflect increasingly accurate, full versions of the "truth" of *reality* and not merely our subjective experiences and beliefs. If we fail to take responsibility for our natural evolutionary predispositions, such as fight-flight-freeze reactivity and immediate gratification and greed tendencies, we will likely not create peace in the world. As material resources meet their limits (for instance, fresh water, rare earth minerals, and energy supplies) and human conflicts continue (such as over limited resources and religious differences), we will be further challenged to create peace. As a result, we need a vision for healthy sustainable living and its accompanying models to unite and guide us on this new path that transports us toward a peaceful, viable future.

Recommendations on the National Level Serve as Guidelines for All Levels

The transformation of society into healthy sustainable living requires integrated, complementary interventions. Each health dimension plays significant roles in moving society toward a viable future. In addition, success depends upon the solution of existing problems and the prevention of anticipated difficulties to complement wellness goals. Therefore, a comprehensive approach that integrates wellness, prevention, and treatment interventions in systematic, progressive ways invites greater success. Additional interventions, appropriate to each level of society and potentially synergistic within and among the different levels, can supplement and extend the effectiveness of these national recommendations. Interventions need prioritized and intentionally synchronized to generate increased effects. These comprehensive tools and methods encourage citizens from all levels of society to work together in pursuit of the common goal to create a healthy sustainable future for the nation and the world.

The Comprehensive and Healthy Living Models Applied to Tobacco Use

I will now propose how to reduce tobacco use with the assistance of the healthy living models. In this case, reductions in tobacco use and healthy living go naturally together. As the number one preventable cause of premature illness and death in the United States, tobacco use appears increasingly manageable when viewed from the comprehensive perspective provided by the healthy living models. In this light, I will present an example of how to integrate the healthy living model and the comprehensive healthy living model in efforts to reduce the use of tobacco across the country.

Initially, the healthy living model provides a systematic means to identify factors that frequently contribute to tobacco use (see Figure 13). This comprehensive assessment of potential causal factors that range across the twelve dimensions of healthy living reveals the complex nature of the problem and shows why simple solutions to tobacco use rarely work. In addition, this screening process facilitates the planning of interventions that confront the underlying causes of tobacco use. Meanwhile, the comprehensive healthy living model facilitates the national and local levels to coordinate planning and intervention efforts. As a result, this comprehensive approach, encompassing different dimensions of health and different levels of society that contribute both to tobacco problems and to their solutions, presents opportunities to confront this deadly problem in increasingly integrated, effective ways.

As the Centers for Disease Control and Prevention (2007a, 7) indicate "evidence-based, statewide tobacco control programs that are comprehensive, sustained, and accountable have been shown to reduce smoking rates, tobacco related death, and diseases caused by smoking." The following use of the comprehensive and the healthy living models provides an example of how to integrate these successful features into a simple, comprehensive format that supports assessment, planning, and coordination of interventions to reduce tobacco use. Simultaneously, these efforts promote the broader goal to develop healthy sustainable living.

To simplify this example, the levels of society have been collapsed into a combined societal component that includes the nation, as well as the state, the community, and the workplace. Accompanying the suggested interventions on the societal level, recommendations on the level of the individual person complement these broader societal interventions. As desired, more specific interventions can be designated on any level within the societal category, such as recommendations directed explicitly to the state or workplace levels.

One in Five Deaths in the United States Is Associated with Smoking

A significant improvement in the health status of the US population depends on our efforts to reduce the use of tobacco among adults and young people. Approximately 443,000 people die each year from tobacco-related illnesses in the nation (Healthy People 2020, 2012). One in every five deaths is smoking-related, according to the Centers for Disease Control and Prevention's Office on Smoking and Health (CDC OSH, 2001). In addition to each person who dies, 20 other people suffer from at least one serious, tobacco-related illness (CDC, 2007a).

Approximately one in five people smoke at this time (CDC, 2009a). In this choice they inadvertently invite great suffering with lung or oral cancers taking their lives, or pulmonary conditions choking off their breathing, or their heart simply stopping. In addition, any secondhand smoke that they spread may sentence some of the people around them to chronic diseases or similar fates.

The estimated medical costs for smoking accumulates to nearly $100 billion annually in the United States, while approximately another $100 billion hurts the economy due to lost productivity. Meanwhile, nearly four thousand adolescents start smoking each day, strongly assisted by the marketing of tobacco companies that spent $13.4 billion in 2005. These companies outspent "the nation's total tobacco prevention and cessation efforts by a ratio of more than 22 to 1" (CDC, 2007a, 32).

Significant numbers of lives, unnecessary suffering, and huge expenses can be saved by stopping smoking. For instance, within several weeks after quitting, lung functions begin to improve and heart attack risk starts to decrease. One year after quitting, the excess risk of heart attack decreases by half, and after fifteen years the risk nearly matches that of a lifelong nonsmoker. Meanwhile, ten years after quitting, the risk of lung cancer death decreases to about half compared to a current smoker (CDC, 2009a).

The Healthy Living Model Differentiates Risk Factors for Smoking

To address this complex and deadly problem that undermines the healthy functioning of society, we first need to understand why people use tobacco products. In this case, the reasons vary for each individual to start smoking. The healthy living model provides a template to identify common reasons or risks that predispose a person to start, and then continue, using tobacco. In the "Healthy Living Model—Smoking Risks" presented in Figure 13, we can efficiently review multi-dimensional risk factors that may contribute to an individual's use of tobacco products.

The risk factors for smoking derive from a multitude of causal possibilities (CDC OSH,

Figure 13:
The Healthy Living Model: Smoking Risks

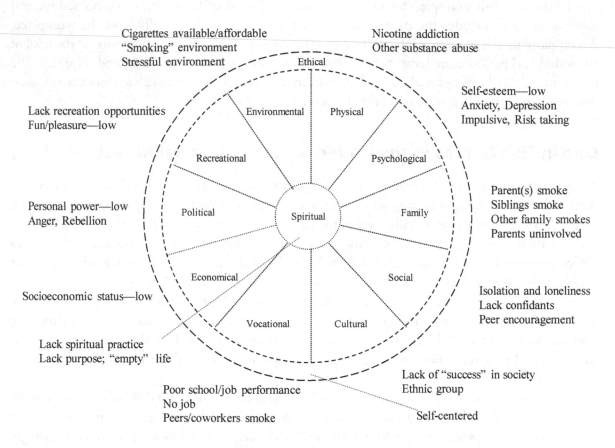

Cigarettes available/affordable
"Smoking" environment
Stressful environment

Nicotine addiction
Other substance abuse

Lack recreation opportunities
Fun/pleasure—low

Self-esteem—low
Anxiety, Depression
Impulsive, Risk taking

Personal power—low
Anger, Rebellion

Parent(s) smoke
Siblings smoke
Other family smokes
Parents uninvolved

Socioeconomic status—low

Isolation and loneliness
Lack confidants
Peer encouragement

Lack spiritual practice
Lack purpose; "empty" life

Poor school/job performance
No job
Peers/coworkers smoke

Lack of "success" in society
Ethnic group

Self-centered

Ethical
Environmental   Physical
Recreational
Psychological
Political   Spiritual   Family
Economical
Social
Vocational   Cultural

1999; 2001; Institute of Medicine, 2000; CDC, 2007a). As indicated in Figure 13, potential risk factors cover the entire healthy living spectrum, as risks arise associated with each of the twelve dimensions. As examples, in the physical dimension, "Other substance abuse," such as alcohol abuse predisposes a person toward tobacco use. Meanwhile, in the psychological dimension, low "Self-esteem," mental health problems, and predispositions to impulsiveness and "Risk taking" contribute to higher use. In the family, social, and cultural dimensions, the encouragement and modeling of other significant people in the person's life increases the probability of tobacco use. "Isolation and loneliness" also increase risk.

In the vocational and economical areas, the lack of opportunities, poor performance, and insufficient rewards for work increase risks for tobacco use. A lack of "personal power" (political), especially accompanied by "anger" and "rebellion," increases the susceptibilities for use. In the recreational and environmental dimensions, the lack of opportunities for fun combined with opportunities to access tobacco products contribute to increased use. Furthermore, the lack of purpose in life (spiritual), and a "self-centered" lifestyle (ethical) can also contribute to the use of tobacco products.

The causes of smoking are complex. A comprehensive approach that considers the multitude of contributors is essential if we intend to realize substantial reductions in tobacco use. Otherwise, when a community addresses certain causal factors (for instance, peer pressure, the lack of recreation, and easy access to affordable tobacco products) but not others (such as low self-esteem and personal power, significant modeling from others that directly or indirectly encourage use, and the lack of success in school, work, home, or the community), the effectiveness of interventions can be limited. The unaddressed causes often continue to motivate people to use tobacco products. As a result, if we intend to succeed in substantially reducing tobacco use, we need to address the multitude of factors that contribute to this costly health problem, ranging from the personal to the societal levels.

The Comprehensive Model Promotes Long-term Solutions to Tobacco Use

The comprehensive healthy living model provides the tools and methodology to organize and coordinate interventions that consider these risk factors, so practical, sustainable solutions can be developed. Figure 14 provides a simplified example of how to use the model to design comprehensive interventions to reduce tobacco use.

For illustration purposes, only two categories of intervention targets will be used—the societal and the individual levels. This means that the societal level collapses the different "Nation/State/Community/Business" levels into one category. Since each of these jurisdictions has particular responsibilities, if needed, these can be portrayed by differentiating the four levels of society into distinct targets and specifying interventions that apply exclusively to each by simply expanding the intervention targets in the model. To simplify this demonstration further, I also collapse the twelve dimensions of health into six major categories of functioning (see Figure 14). For instance, the vocational and economical areas become the "work/money" health dimension.

Figure 14:
Comprehensive Healthy Living Interventions to Reduce Tobacco Use

Types of Interventions

Intervention Target: Nation/State/Community/Workplace

Health Dimensions	Wellness	Prevention	Treatment
Physical Body	Develop Healthy Sustainable Living (HSL) practices to decrease risks in all 12 areas	Develop health insurance that covers comprehensive preventive services	Implement insurance coverage that pays for smoking cessation
Psychological	Teach HSL practices through schools, workplaces, and the media, including social media	Support the development of life skills for the general public over their lifespan	Integrated tobacco cessation programs—"quitline" + support + counseling + medications
Social/Cultural	Develop partnerships for HSL to change social norms and coordinate programs/policies	Provide media campaigns regarding dangers of tobacco use and second-hand smoke	Comprehensive treatment that addresses causal factors in the 12 HL dimensions (see Figure 13)
Work/Money	Fund comprehensive tobacco control programs	Increase and use tobacco taxes to help pay for these interventions	Employ policies/legislation to use tobacco fines and law suits to pay for these interventions
Environmental	Develop surveillance and evaluation accountability	Develop policies/legislation for tobacco-free environments and enforcement	Increase taxes and fines on tobacco products
Spiritual/Ethical	Develop and model ethics and spiritual practices consistent with HSL	Research how tobacco use detracts from HSL, and calculate the economic costs	Implement spiritual, HSL treatments for tobacco users

Intervention Target: Individual

Health Dimensions	Wellness	Prevention	Treatment
Physical Body	Develop healthy exercise, nutrition, relaxation habits	Avoid substance abuse in any form	Enroll in a comprehensive smoking cessation program—counseling + support + meds
Psychological	Use healthy living, self-esteem building, and assertiveness practices	Redirect risk-taking behaviors into non-lethal, non-destructive alternatives	Treat anxiety, depression, and impulse-control issues
Social/Cultural	Develop social support systems that promote no tobacco use	Avoid tobacco if family members/friends smoke	Seek treatment with supportive peers; increase health care education/referrals
Work/Money	Utilize and support healthy sustainable living programs in work/school	Choose not to work for a company that sells or promotes tobacco use	Encourage and support tobacco users to quit
Environmental	Develop lifestyles aligned with healthy, tobacco-free environments	Support the development of tobacco-free environments	Help enforce tobacco control measures and assertiveness regarding second-hand smoke
Spiritual/Ethical	Implement a spiritual practice	Volunteer to serve others and the world	Develop meditation or contemplation skills

With the model simplified for demonstration purposes, I will now highlight several recommendations of interventions that can be directed toward the nation/state/community/business and the individual levels of society. These recommendations will be applied across the six composite dimensions of health.

Nation/State/Community/Business Interventions

The first recommendation described under "Types of Interventions" in Figure 14 involves the wellness area. This recommendation applies to the nation/state/community/business levels of society as the "Intervention Target." Meanwhile, the "Health Dimensions" category designates the physical body as the recipient of the intervention. In this context, the initial recommendation in the upper left cell of the table focuses on the priority to "Develop healthy sustainable living (HSL) practices" to decrease the risks of tobacco use across all twelve dimensions of potential contributions.

Since tobacco use arises from a combination of risk factors distributed throughout the twelve dimensions, the optimal way to decrease the risk of tobacco use involves the development of healthy lifestyles. Such lifestyles depend on the development of conscious awareness to choose how to overcome the influences presented by the risk factors. In this case, we need conscious choices that select healthy behaviors to replace unhealthy behaviors and reactive patterns that lead to tobacco use.

The wellness and prevention options associated with the psychological dimension support healthy skill development. These skills include healthy living practices taught in schools, workplaces, and through the media, including the social media. Through these education programs that reach across the lifespan, we progressively learn the skills necessary to achieve our overarching goal for healthy sustainable living. As we learn these skills, we can work to overcome the risk factors often associated with tobacco use (see figure 13).

In the wellness social/cultural area, we can "Develop partnerships" between national, state, and local governments, as well as organizations, businesses, and private citizens. Such partnerships can combine efforts to control tobacco use and improve healthy living. Cooperative partnerships can promote changes in social norms and behaviors while accelerating the development of healthy living on multiple levels of society.

Wellness in the "Work/Money" arena requires adequate funding for comprehensive tobacco control programs. Such funding can come from tobacco taxes, fines, and law suits, so the people and corporations that profit from tobacco products can pay for the interventions necessary to repair part of the resultant damages. For instance, medical expenses and lost productivity alone amount to about $200 billion a year. These cumulative costs, however, depend on measurements in the costs of tobacco use in only about one third of the dimensions that make up healthy living. This means that psychological, family, social, environmental, and ethical costs, for instance, largely go unnoticed and still not quantified.

Therefore, in the prevention "Spiritual/Ethical" area, the recommendation is to identify the problems and suffering generated, then calculate the costs of tobacco use to individuals and to all levels of society throughout the twelve healthy living dimensions. In this way, a more accurate accounting of the extensive costs associated with tobacco use can be identified.

Accountability and surveillance need incorporated into efforts to reduce tobacco use, as indicated in the wellness "Environmental" area. For instance, monitoring of "tobacco-related attitudes, behaviors, and health outcomes at regular intervals" (CDC, 2007a, 9) enables the effectiveness of different interventions to be evaluated, so we continually improve our planning efforts. As suggested in the wellness, spiritual/ethical recommendation, reductions in tobacco use depend on people developing and modeling healthy sustainable living practices. For instance, the service providers in the tobacco reduction efforts need to model tobacco-free lifestyles to emulate the desired social norms.

The other recommendations for interventions on the nation/state/community/business level seem relatively self-explanatory, with the exception of the final recommendation in the treatment spiritual/ethical category. In this case, efforts to "Implement spiritual, HSL treatments for tobacco users" means that service providers initially screen for the underlying reasons the person started and continues to use tobacco, based on the risk factors affiliated with the twelve dimensions of the healthy living model. By understanding the motivations and cues that support the use of tobacco across these dimensions, interventions can be specifically tailored to help each person break the habit by replacing old behaviors and beliefs with new healthy ones.

To complement these interventions and assist the person to eliminate or manage risk factors, the spiritual dimension provides other valuable resources. For instance, spiritually based psychotherapy serves to help people transcend their addictive patterns. Along these lines, we enjoy three types of existence: mortal, immortal, and eternal. Addictions arise primarily from perceptions and functions based on our mortal nature. Meanwhile, our immortal and eternal natures can help us transcend the problems that we create on the mortal level. The immortal and eternal natures also help fill the spiritual emptiness often associated with addictions.

Individual Interventions

The "Individual" serves as a natural target for interventions in order to reduce the use of tobacco. Comprehensive interventions on the individual level range across the same six health dimensions categories used for the societal interventions. Since these recommendations generally attempt to overcome specific risk factors associated with tobacco use, they seem relatively straightforward compared to the more complex, policy interventions on the nation/state/community/business level. While this example provides insight into how the healthy living models can help solve complex human problems, a more complete list of specific intervention targets to reduce tobacco use may also include the family, social, workplace and school levels of society. Since each of these levels often influence the use of tobacco, focused interventions into these areas can also contribute solutions to treat, prevent, and transcend this deadly problem.

Summary

This example demonstrates how the combination of the healthy living model and the comprehensive healthy living model provides an integrated methodology that can be used to help solve any human problem. The integrated methodology of assessment, planning, and comprehensive interventions, followed naturally by evaluations of the results, can lead to an ongoing feedback system that can progressively solve problems and simultaneously enhance healthy living. These two models synergize to promote healthy solutions to the problems that we face in the world, as they also contribute to the larger vision to improve healthy sustainable living for individuals, the society, and the global community.

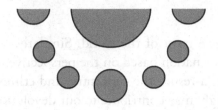

CHAPTER 9

The Ethical Living Model Supports Evolution and Prevents Devolution

• • • • • • •

A healthy sustainable future depends on our living in harmony with *reality*. To create harmonious living requires that we evaluate how our actions affect the different levels of the world upon which our lives depend. Such a comprehensive evaluation requires that we develop a standardized method that people throughout the world can use and through which we perceive all the major dimensions and levels of *reality* necessary for sustainability.

The Ethical Living Model portrays these crucial dimensions and levels necessary for sustainability (see Figure 15). The model enables us to identify both short-term benefits and costs (see Figure 16), and potential devolutionary outcomes from our actions, as well as evolutionary actions we can initiate for health and sustainability (see Figure 17). Each level in the model needs to function as well as interact productively across the levels to support sustainable living. The twelve dimensions of the healthy living model function on each of the societal levels. These dimensions operate universally within each and across all levels as they interact to form healthy living. In combination, healthy living across all these societal levels produces the foundation for sustainable living.

The Evolutionary Ethical Living Model

The ethical living model portrays universal functioning, as it provides an overview of *reality*. The healthy living dimensions apply across all levels of society and simultaneously impact all levels of evolution. Evolutionary form arises from the ground of being as spiritual evolution in which the infinite potential of spirit manifests into evolutionary form. This combination of human, evolutionary, and spiritual functioning produces a comprehensive overview of both our presence and our participation in *reality*. This inclusive perspective introduces a standardized tool from which we can evaluate how our actions contribute to the evolution or the devolution of humanity, the planet, and *reality*.

Typically, we initiate actions with the intent of contributing to evolution. Nevertheless, when we perceive only those aspects of *reality* that pertain to our self at the egocentric level of consciousness, we fail to perceive most of the world. Similarly, when we attempt to evolve on behalf of our family, business, or nation based on the perspective of ethnocentric consciousness, we still omit most of *reality*. As a result, the egocentric and ethnocentric perspectives serve our special interests, yet unknowingly may contribute to our devolution.

For example, when we accidentally harm the levels of society and levels of evolution that exist beyond our awareness, we unsuspectingly undermine our lives. Since long-term satisfaction of our interests depends upon the functioning of all these supporting levels of existence, we must protect all these levels from devolutionary outcomes. Otherwise, we may contribute to our evolution in the short-term by satisfying our special interests while unknowingly contributing to our long-term devolution.

The ethical living model portrays the "Self" at the top of Figure 15. We stand upon all levels of *reality* that have developed prior to us and that actually support our existence. Yet when we perceive this figure through egocentric eyes, we commonly perceive our self as the most important part of the figure. Sometimes we even perceive that the universe exists to serve our needs as we stand at the top or at the center of it all.

In contrast, from an evolutionary perspective the individual self exists on the surface layer, actually dependent on and therefore responsible to all these deeper levels. These levels that support humanity ("Family, Workplace, Community, Nation, World") and, more significantly, all the levels of evolution ("Cultural, Human, Biological, Physical, Spiritual") symbolize our social self and evolutionary self that enable our individual self to exist. Devolutionary harm to any of these levels of society and evolution fundamentally shakes our foundation and can result in our individual death—and ultimately in the demise of all humanity.

The Vision for Healthy Sustainable Living Depends on our Perceptions of Reality

We must develop methods to perceive beyond the limitations of our egocentric and ethnocentric perspectives (dominant among 70 percent of people in the world) if we intend to create a healthy sustainable future for humanity. The ethical living model presents a simplified version of a kosmocentric viewpoint. In other words, the model portrays aspects of *reality* that exist beyond and too complex for normal human awareness. It introduces the opportunity to experience a temporary state of consciousness in which we can perceive more fully and accurately than available from our normal egocentric, ethnocentric, or even worldcentric viewpoints.

The inclusive view of *reality* provided by the ethical living model enables us to evaluate how our actions may generate evolutionary and devolutionary consequences that occur beyond our special interest concerns. Thus, we can evaluate the potential ramifications of our cocreative efforts as they ripple throughout all levels of existence. We can now begin to assess both the evolutionary and devolutionary consequences of our actions before we act. The ultimate ethical choice emerges: "Do our consciousness and actions contribute to evolution or to devolution?" With this ethical perspective, healthy sustainable living emerges as a viable option for humanity to pursue.

Figure 15:
The Ethical Living Model

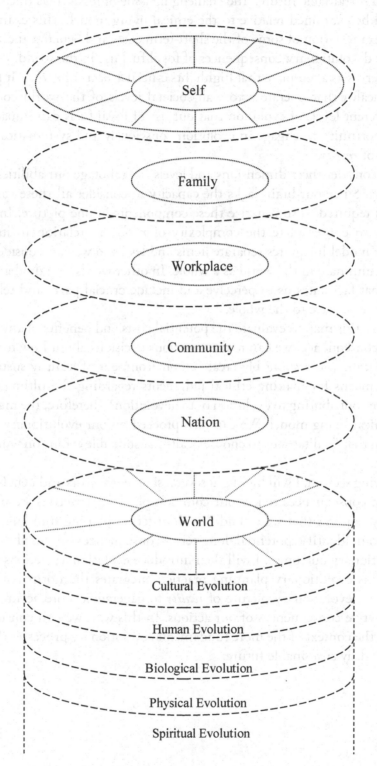

Self

Family

Workplace

Community

Nation

World

Cultural Evolution

Human Evolution

Biological Evolution

Physical Evolution

Spiritual Evolution

The Ethical Living Model—Applied to the Use of Fossil Fuels

The remainder of the chapter will provide a demonstration of how the model can help us assess how to develop a sustainable future. The challenging issue of fossil fuels (including oil, coal, and natural gas) will be examined relative to the ethical living model. This example will provide a comprehensive examination of some of the short-term costs and benefits and, more importantly, the potential for devolutionary consequences of fossil fuel use in the world.

The model serves as a template that highlights crucial aspects of *reality*. It portrays the twelve dimensions of health that operate across all societal levels of the world community and also includes the different levels of evolution that our use of fossil fuels can impact. The model also presents the opportunity to engage in evolution consciously and systematically across all levels and dimensions of *reality*.

If we fail to consider these dimensions and levels, we sabotage our abilities to pursue healthy sustainable living. Since our brain lacks the capacity to consider all these variables at the same time, a model is required to summarize these components in one picture. In this way, we have the opportunity to contemplate the complexity of *reality* in relation to its many levels and dimensions. The model integrates separate items and levels so we can consider the relationships that ultimately culminate in the world as a whole. In other words, the model represents a simple map of *reality* that facilitates us to perceive and include crucial parts and relationships that we consider important relative to the whole.

We can utilize this map to evaluate the potential costs and benefits of any action throughout the world. As a consequence, we can make conscious decisions about how to promote evolution instead of devolution and responsibly create an environment of healthy sustainable living. The map provides a means for making ethical judgments regarding the ultimate dynamics in the universe—are we contributing to evolution or to devolution? Therefore, the map can be called the evolutionary ethical living model. We can now proceed on our evolutionary journey guided by an ethical system that facilitates us to choose healthy sustainable evolution while we intentionally avoid devolution.

In the following section, I will highlight several short-term costs and benefits of fossil fuel use. These short-term consequences reflect our common planning practices we use today. Planning for sustainability requires that we extend this short-term planning into long-term evolutionary planning. We can identify potential long-term consequences of fossil fuel use, including potential devolutionary outcomes. I will then introduce evolutionary actions to move us toward sustainability. This evolutionary planning practice integrates the normal short-term planning perspective into an evolutionary picture of *reality* to generate a more accurate portrayal of the positive and negative consequences of our actions. In this way, we can consider our immediate concerns within the context of the more fundamental evolutionary processes that hold the secrets to achieving a healthy sustainable future.

Short-Term Costs Associated with the Use of Fossil Fuels

Self and Family Levels

The short-term costs of the use of fossil fuels occur across all levels of the ethical living model. Figure 16 provides examples of both the short-term costs and the short-term benefits of fossil fuel use. Initially, the costs will be discussed, followed in the next section by the benefits. The first example of short-term costs experienced on the individual or "Self" level involves increases in the price of gasoline and consumer goods whenever shortages of fossil fuels occur. Similarly, price increases in the areas of food, utilities, transportation, and services represent common expenses experienced on the "Family" or household level when fuel shortages occur.

Business Level

In the "Business" section, for instance, fossil fuel shortages associated with oil embargoes and electrical grid shutdowns can result in cost increases and production decreases to goods and services. The costs of fossil fuel use in the workplace dramatically increase when the costs to people and the planet are included. Normally, human and environment costs are considered as externalities, without quantifiable monetary value in economic terms. For instance, the price of coal increases four to five times when several of the human and environmental costs are included in its price (Yarra Valley Climate Action Group, 2012).

Community Level

Costs on the local "Community" level can involve smog, acid rain, water pollution, and the depletion of freshwater supplies due to fossil fuel use. In addition, communities associated with energy extraction and production can experience sudden booms and busts in their population when demands for energy change. For instance, human service caseloads dramatically rise when rapid increases in the population of rural energy communities occur. A 100 percent increase in the population of rural energy communities has been found to result in disproportionate demands for human services, including mental health—286 percent; alcohol—414 percent; chemical abuse—314 percent; domestic violence—210 percent; rape—233 percent; youth disturbances—314 percent; income maintenance—210 percent; and social services—210 percent (Department of the Air Force, 1984). Similarly, when the "Boom" ends and the community goes "Bust," social, psychological, and additional economic stresses occur that can also lead to disproportionate human service demands.

Figure 16:
The Ethical Living Model: Short-term Costs and Benefits of Fossil Fuels

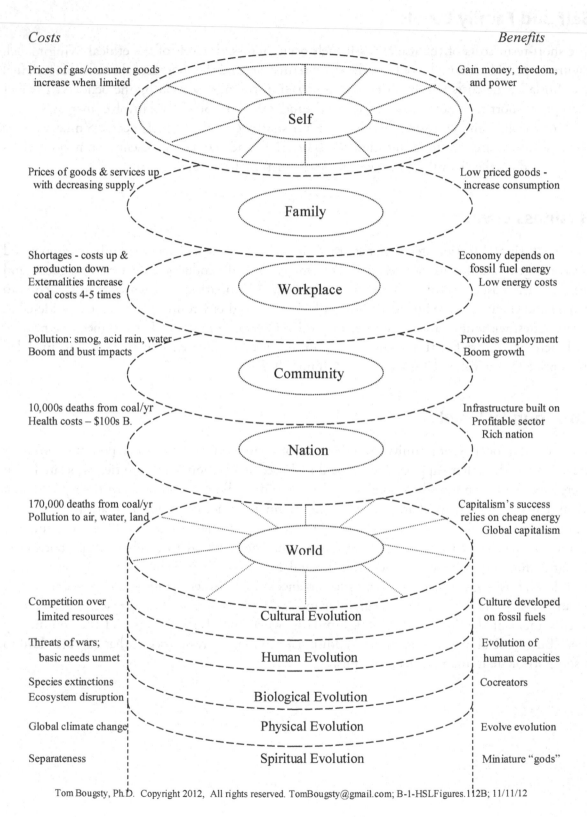

Costs   *Benefits*

Prices of gas/consumer goods
increase when limited

Gain money, freedom,
and power

Self

Prices of goods & services up
with decreasing supply

Low priced goods -
increase consumption

Family

Shortages - costs up &
production down
Externalities increase
coal costs 4-5 times

Economy depends on
fossil fuel energy
Low energy costs

Workplace

Pollution: smog, acid rain, water
Boom and bust impacts

Provides employment
Boom growth

Community

10,000s deaths from coal/yr
Health costs – $100s B.

Infrastructure built on
Profitable sector
Rich nation

Nation

170,000 deaths from coal/yr
Pollution to air, water, land

Capitalism's success
relies on cheap energy
Global capitalism

World

Competition over
limited resources

Cultural Evolution

Culture developed
on fossil fuels

Threats of wars;
basic needs unmet

Human Evolution

Evolution of
human capacities

Species extinctions
Ecosystem disruption

Biological Evolution

Cocreators

Global climate change

Physical Evolution

Evolve evolution

Separateness

Spiritual Evolution

Miniature "gods"

Nation Level

Pollution from coal-burning power plants causes tens of thousands of deaths per year and hundreds of billions of dollars of health care costs in the United States. In efforts to remediate these problems, the Cross-State Air Pollution Rule by the Environmental Protection Agency intends to reduce this pollution. The anticipated results of reductions in coal pollution include saving from 13,000 to 34,000 premature deaths and saving from $120 to $280 billion in health care and environmental costs by 2014, as well as each year thereafter (US Environmental Protection Agency, 2012).

World Level

The vast majority of the energy use in the world derives from fossil fuels. Hence, high rates of death and health care costs similarly result on the global level. For instance, pollutants from coal-based electricity minimally kill 170,000 people annually (Polya, 2008). Damages occur, usually unmeasured in monetary costs, to the air, water, and land environments of Earth as continued extraction, production, distribution, disposal, and pollution from fossil fuels proceeds.

Cultural and Human Evolution Levels

Meanwhile, when we consider the "Cultural" level of evolution, the competition for these desirable, finite fossil fuel resources continues to increase. Since the global economy depends on these limited fossil fuels, nations compete, sometimes suffer shortages, and even go to war over resource conflicts. On the "Human" level of evolution, wars related to energy resources threaten our future. Similarly, insufficient energy resources can lead to suffering and death from shortages of food, water, and industrial production of goods and services necessary for life.

Biological, Physical, and Spiritual Evolution Levels

On the "Biological" level of evolution, a variety of side effects from fossil fuel use include dramatic increases in the extinction of animal and plant species, as well as increasing acidification of waterways and the oceans that provide sources for human food. Complex ecosystems upon which all life depends suffer increasing damage and disruptions. Meanwhile, on the "Physical" level of evolution, we continue to burn fossil fuels as our main source of energy production despite the nonrenewable and polluting qualities of these resources. Global climate change results with increases in destructive weather events, such as floods, wildfires, droughts, and severe storms. Destructive weather accompanied by rising ocean levels and other unpredictable changes threaten our future. From the "Spiritual" level, since we perceive fossil fuels and the world largely through the separateness lens, we fail to perceive our interconnected, interdependent oneness with all *reality*. Hence, our natural relationships with our collective humanity and with all nature typically remain beyond our awareness. We can then naïvely exploit these relationships and the oneness of all in attempts to satisfy our short-term needs and desires.

Short-Term Benefits Associated with the Use of Fossil Fuels

Self and Family Levels

Fossil fuels enable our "Self" to enjoy the conveniences of modern life. When adequate supplies of energy exist, job opportunities to make money can give us the power to meet our basic needs. With the satisfaction of these needs, we experience the freedom to shift our attention to other lifestyle choices. For example on the "Family" level, when basic needs for heating, cooling, and electricity in our homes are met, we experience the freedom to consume other goods produced from fossil fuels, such as clothes, medications, and plastic products. Since the cost of fossil fuels excludes most of the human and planetary costs as externalities, the price of goods and services are kept artificially low, thereby promoting the consumption of goods and services. Consumer purchases account for 70 percent of the economic output in the United States (Leeb, 2009), and thereby, consumer consumption serves as the primary driver of the economy.

Business Level

Since fossil fuels have traditionally been relatively easy to find, cheap to produce, and represent a stable, fairly efficient energy source, they provide the surplus energy needed to grow the economy. Beyond human energy, fossil fuels supply the bulk of the energy to expand the economy. For instance, these fuels provide the energy to construct the infrastructure, industrial development, and technologies that generate consumer goods and services that grow the economy. In a sense, fossil fuels function like a treasure chest that we have discovered and convert into low cost energy to power our lives and grow the economy.

Community and Nation Levels

On the "Community" level, employment opportunities arise from the technological and industrial development that fossil fuel energy helps generate. When demands for fossil fuels increase, rapid growth experienced as "Booms" in energy resource communities can result in significant population growth and revenues for the local area. The fundamental infrastructure of the "Nation" exists as a result of the energy produced from fossil fuels. The energy industry that supplies these fuels operates as one of the most profitable sectors in the economy. The cheap energy provided by fossil fuels empowers growth in the economy, generates significant profits for many corporations, and helps create an economically rich nation. In many ways, the success of the nation stands on the use of fossil fuels.

World, Cultural, and Human Evolution Levels

The combination of capitalism and fossil fuels has produced so many successes that they have been adopted as the methods to create success throughout much of the world. Historically, fossil fuels appear as the natural resource to lead the "World" into the future. Capitalism serves as the economic system in which fossil fuels operate as an inexpensive resource from which economic growth and material development can satisfy our needs and pleasures. Thus, "Cultural" evolution has been significantly influenced by fossil fuels. Their continued use appears as the obvious path to follow to perpetuate our past successes into a future of growth and prosperity. Thus, the economic development and modernization of the world depends on cheap available fossil fuels.

"Human" evolution that expands our consciousness and creativity has soared as a side benefit of fossil fuel use. We now generate more change in the world than traditional random mutations produce. We have expanded the life expectancies of individuals and dramatically increased the human population throughout the world. Fossil fuels have provided the surplus energy that frees us to develop our cognitive and creative capacities, so we function increasingly as an evolutionary force in the world.

Biological, Physical, and Spiritual Evolution Levels

Fossil fuels have supplied the surplus energy that enables humans to transform nature. For example, technologies have been developed to expand food production through mechanized farming, irrigation, and genetic manipulation. "Biological" and "Physical" evolution both change as we act like cocreators in service to our needs and desires. In the process, we evolve evolution. From the "Spiritual" perspective, humans have developed into seeming "miniature gods" who capture the energy from millions of years of past generations of life to transform the world in our own image.

Devolution—Long-Term Costs Associated with the Use of Fossil Fuels

Devolution—Self and Family Levels

Fossil fuels have dominated the energy arena for nearly two centuries. Their relatively inexpensive and accessible nature has provided humans with an opportunity to evolve at accelerated rates regarding industrial and cultural development. In this successful process, we have inadvertently become dependent on, or unsuspectingly addicted to, fossil fuels to maintain and grow our present lifestyles.

Beyond our dependence on fossil fuels, capitalism has reinforced that private interests represent the legitimate means to develop, process, distribute, and work with this evolutionary store of fossil fuel energy. Hence, capitalism institutionalized private interests as the means to develop the economy. Egocentric, self-centered lifestyles naturally followed, as seen in the "Self" level of society depicted in the ethical living model (see Figure 17). When self-interests extend into group interests on the "Family" through the "Nation" levels of society, we shift from egocentric into ethnocentric consciousness. In this process, capitalism has institutionalized private, special interests of the self and the group (for instance, family, corporation, and nation), as more important than public, collective interests of humanity and the planet.

As discussed previously, both egocentric and ethnocentric levels of consciousness lack adequate awareness of *reality* from which to create a sustainable future. Hence, our fossil fuel dependence, supported by our capitalist economy, unsuspectingly supports our conscious development to operate

Figure 17:
The Ethical Living Model: Long-term Devolution Costs of Fossil Fuels and Health and Sustainability Benefits from Evolutionary Planning and Actions

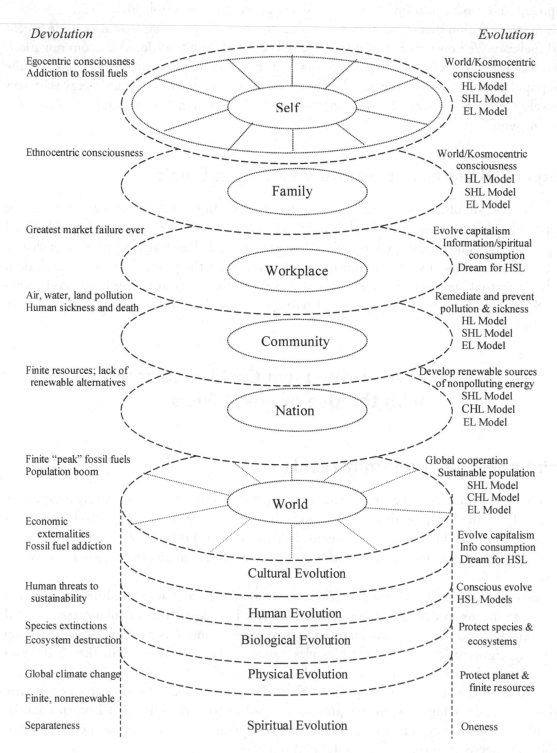

Devolution

Egocentric consciousness
Addiction to fossil fuels

Ethnocentric consciousness

Greatest market failure ever

Air, water, land pollution
Human sickness and death

Finite resources; lack of
renewable alternatives

Finite "peak" fossil fuels
Population boom

Economic
externalities
Fossil fuel addiction

Human threats to
sustainability

Species extinctions
Ecosystem destruction

Global climate change

Finite, nonrenewable

Separateness

Evolution

World/Kosmocentric
consciousness
HL Model
SHL Model
EL Model

World/Kosmocentric
consciousness
HL Model
SHL Model
EL Model

Evolve capitalism
Information/spiritual
consumption
Dream for HSL

Remediate and prevent
pollution & sickness
HL Model
SHL Model
EL Model

Develop renewable sources
of nonpolluting energy
SHL Model
CHL Model
EL Model

Global cooperation
Sustainable population
SHL Model
CHL Model
EL Model

Evolve capitalism
Info consumption
Dream for HSL

Conscious evolve
HSL Models

Protect species &
ecosystems

Protect planet &
finite resources

Oneness

Self

Family

Workplace

Community

Nation

World

Cultural Evolution

Human Evolution

Biological Evolution

Physical Evolution

Spiritual Evolution

at unsustainable, self-destructive levels. Furthermore, since individual and group consumption and production primarily serve personal and group interests, harm to other people and the planet often goes undetected or appears unimportant from a private interest viewpoint. The damages to people and the planet that result from our self-centered and group-centered pursuits sometimes undermine the life-support systems necessary for our survival.

Devolution—Business Level

On the "Business" level, the use of fossil fuels presents the potential for the greatest market failure ever. Fossil fuels, in conjunction with the six following limitations embedded in the capitalist economic system, provide the match that may ignite a global market meltdown.

Assumptions Associated with Capitalism Need to Evolve

The capitalist economic system appears endangered by several of its own basic assumptions. These assumptions and their associated economic activities need to evolve to make capitalism and, more importantly, humanity sustainable. For instance, the system has proven so successful due to assumptions that seemed appropriate in past centuries. These conventions, accompanied by the evolutionary gift of living organisms dying and decomposing to form fossil fuels, power our economy. Yet these millions of years of life result in only finite quantities of fossil fuels to burn for our energy consumption. These fuels, and our inadvertent addiction to them, have enabled us to have the surplus energy to power our creative construction of modern society. However, the depletion of our finite "drug of choice" places us and the economy in an untenable position regarding devolutionary risks to humanity and the planet, unless we invest in and discover affordable, nonpolluting, and renewable sources of energy.

The following assumptions associated with the capitalist system align partially with *reality* (see chapter 6) but not fully enough to lead to a sustainable future. Moreover, many of these assumptions make it easier to perpetuate our addiction to fossil fuels that further increases the likelihood that we will experience a global market failure.

- *Value*: Money determines value, yet money cannot be easily applied to complex living systems like humans and the environment that are essential to our existence. As a result, people and the planet are often converted into externalities with little or no measurable value, and therefore, can be unintentionally or intentionally exploited for monetary profits and material consumption. Fossil fuels represent a prime example of people and the planet being treated as externalities. Despite the threat of devolutionary harm to both humans and the environment (for instance, through global climate change, ozone depletion, and potential wars), fossil fuels continue as a cheap source of energy that holds the elite position as the fuel to power the world economy. Thus, the value system of the capitalist economy only partially, and sometimes inaccurately, reflects *reality*, and consequently, propels us towards devolution.

- *Process*: Material objects, such as fossil fuels, are fundamental to the sustenance of the economy and money measures the success of its development. Consequently, the lens of separateness dominates and limits our perceptions of *reality*, promotes consumption and addictions to these finite resources, and unknowingly leads toward an unsustainable future.

- *Goal*: Growth occurs primarily through material consumption that relies significantly on diminishing resources like fossil fuels that lack the availability for sustainable growth. Despite diminishing fossil fuel resources, many of the most profitable corporations in the world operate in the fossil fuel industry.

- *Motivation*: Competition functions as the designated driver of the economy resulting in winners and losers, haves and have-nots, and simultaneously undermines cooperation and trust necessary for sustainability. Fossil fuel corporations compete so well that they have gained disproportionate influence within the society.

- *Rights*: Private, special interests prioritize individuals and corporations as the most important participants in the economy. This reinforces our natural special interest orientation in which egocentric and ethnocentric views make us appear at the center of *reality*. Such self- and group-centered perspectives lead to actions that eventually generate unsustainable outcomes for the whole of humanity and the planet. In this case, corporations related to fossil fuels have special interest rights to make profits that appear as more important than the collective interests of the public and the planet that face catastrophic long-term consequences from the pollution generated by this source of energy.

- *Power*: Authoritarian styles of management and hierarchical business models, accompanied by authoritative decision making, exclude most democratic, cooperative participation in economic decisions. The power enabled by these previous assumptions gives special interest rights to compete and grow profits through the development of finite nonrenewable material resources that remain cheap due to externalizing long-term costs onto the health of people and the planet. Despite the desperate need for alternative fuels, the power accrued by the fossil fuel industry can be seen by more subsidies still going to the development of fossil fuels than subsidies for the development of new sustainable fuels. In contrast, global cooperation instead of competition will be required to manage the forthcoming shortages anticipated for fossil fuels. Such cooperation can create opportunities to develop a healthy global economy and, more importantly, a sustainable world for humanity.

These assumptions of the capitalist system unsuspectingly lead corporations, the society, and the world to support economic development that leads us toward an unsustainable future. As we continue to rely on finite fossil fuels to drive the world economy, shortages of these fuels will increasingly expose these limitations embedded in the economic system. For example, if the demands for energy exceed supplies, then disruptions to industrial production, financial markets, and the means to meet basic human needs can suddenly occur. Threats to our basic needs often appear as threats to our lives. Under such conditions we react naturally to save our lives and livelihoods. The evolutionary predisposition to react with fight, flight, and freeze reactions has the potential to precipitate cycles of violence and destruction. In a world in which we have developed weapons of mass destruction such human reactivity can light the fuse that burns toward our devolution. In this case, shortages of fossil fuels provide the symbolic match with which to light this devolutionary fuse.

For instance, the goal of growth will suddenly be unsustainable due to the limits of these finite, fossil fuel resources. Despite the efforts of special interests, competition, money expenditures, and authoritarian efforts to achieve economic growth again, the finite limits of these energy resources will likely ignite a financial meltdown that can lead to the greatest market failure ever. More importantly, such a meltdown may initiate a vicious devolutionary cycle.

As other examples of the risk of an economic market failure, Chris Martenson (Daly, Martenson, Fitz-Gerald, and Moors, 2012) says, "To maintain our current way of life, the so-called American Dream, we have to rely on the false belief that we can preserve exponential growth forever in three systems, Energy, the Environment, and the Economy." Since energy and many other environmental resources exist in finite supplies, exponential growth cannot be maintained in any of these three systems. As a result, the authors conclude that we now stand on the verge of economic collapse.

Devolution—Community Level

The "Community" level can experience a variety of pollutants from fossil fuels that harm the local residents and the surrounding environment. These damages include air pollution in the form of smog, ozone, and acid rain; water pollution and depletion; and land degradation in the excavation of natural areas, as well as from accidental spills of fossil fuels. Human damages range from death and illness as a result of fossil fuel pollution to the stresses associated with their extraction, production, use, disposal, pollution, and finite existence.

Devolution—Nation Level

The economy depends on fossil fuels to drive economic growth in the "Nation." Unfortunately, fossil fuels are finite resources that appear increasingly incapable of meeting our demands. Due to their finite nature, they are simply insufficient to create a sustainable future. Diminishing supplies of these vital resources convert the world into a potential tinderbox. As supplies diminish, competition will increase for these valued, but limited resources. Competition generates winners and losers in recreational games, but in the real world, losers sometimes take the form of bankrupt corporations or worse—the death of people. In the world of modern weaponry and terrorism, special interest competition for fossil fuels threatens our ability to create a healthy sustainable future.

Despite the limited nature of fossil fuels, we have failed to develop adequate alternative energy sources to replace the crucial role that fossil fuels play. For instance, in the United States in 2009, only 8 percent of our energy needs were met by the use of renewable energy sources, including water (hydroelectric); geothermal (heat generated and stored in the Earth) ; wind; sun (solar); and biomass (energy from biological organisms) (EIA, 2010). On the global level, 10 percent of energy needs in 2008 were met by renewable sources, while forecasts for 2035 show only 14 percent of total world energy consumption to be met by renewable sources (EIA, 2010).

As can be seen, we have substantially failed to plan and implement how to replace these finite resources with renewable energy. Furthermore, instead of decreasing our greenhouse gas emissions, we have mostly increased them in the United States since 1990 at about 1 percent per year (EIA, 2011). In 2005, about 21 percent of the world's total energy-related carbon dioxide was emitted by the United States. Of these greenhouse gas emissions, 87 percent came from fossil fuel energy consumption. Thus, our addictive use of fossil fuels nudges the United States, as well as the rest of the world, toward devolution, despite the evolutionary gains that accompany the use of these fuels.

Devolution—World Level

On the "World" scene, finite resources mean supplies will diminish while demands likely increase, causing prices to increase as well. Since all the fossil fuels—oil, coal, and natural gas—are finite resources, a peak in their extraction will occur. This means that after the maximum rate of extraction occurs, the resources will progressively decline in their accessibility. Their economic costs will dramatically increase as supplies fail to meet demands. In addition, pollution associated with their extraction, processing, and disposal will also likely increase.

The peak in the discovery of oil occurred in the 1960s. In 1981, the world used more oil than it discovered in new fields (Campbell, 2009). More recently, oil has been consumed at four times the rate that new discoveries have been found (Peak Oil, 2009). Many countries have already passed their peak in oil production suggesting that the peak in world production is "imminent" (Campbell, 2009).

Consequences of Peak Oil

When demands for oil outstrip supplies, major changes may occur, such as:

- Substantial spikes in prices can be expected. For instance, during the oil shocks in the 1970s, "shortfalls in production as small as 5 percent caused the price of oil to nearly quadruple. The same thing happened in California a few years ago with natural gas: a production drop of less than 5 percent caused prices to skyrocket by 400 percent" (http://www.lifeaftertheoilcrash.net/, 2009).

- Modern societies based on complex systems of electricity, transportation, industrial production, and agriculture may collapse, not from running out of oil but from lacking sufficient oil at appropriate times to keep these interconnected systems functioning and working as an interdependent whole (http://www.lifeaftertheoilcrash.net/, 2009).

- Financial markets can then be expected to crash.

Since shortfalls in supplies will begin and increasingly occur, the effects on the financial system may be severe. To place this in a historical context, Campbell (2009) explains that cheap and abundant fossil fuels changed the world of industry, transportation, trade, and agriculture while enabling the global population to increase six-fold (another exponential, unsustainable growth curve). Fossil fuel use provided the necessary source of energy to drive this growth. However, even minor shortfalls in the supplies of fossil fuels have resulted in dramatic price increases in the past. When significant shortfalls actually block the functioning of a critical pillar of the modern economy, catastrophic consequences may result.

Exponential Growth in Debt Undermines our Sustainability

Campbell indicated that rapid growth in financial capital also occurred as banks lent more money than they had on deposit. Seemingly, they could lend more than they possessed because the expanding surpluses in energy created by fossil fuels appeared to assure future growth. The growth in fossil fuel energy introduced a sense of insurance that economic growth would continue despite its short-term volatility. This perspective that long-term growth would persevere seemed to diminish the risk involved in short-term lending, and thereby, the economy had the capital to grow at accelerated rates.

The following provides an example of how the economic system supports exponential growth in our debt. Martenson explains that regulations for financial institutions developed to allow banks to lend 90 percent of their deposits, meaning that an actual $1,000 deposit can turn into $10,000 in "fake money" when multiple banks progressively lend this money (Daly, Martenson, Fitz-Gerald, and Moors, 2012). Therefore, the total credit market debt when we "loan money into existence" grows exponentially and threatens the economy with overwhelming debt. For example, indebtedness of a family of four in the United States amounts to about $691,000, and it continues to grow exponentially.

As the finite nature of fossil fuels that power the economy becomes more widely accepted, the belief that growth will continue indefinitely becomes increasingly in doubt. Without assurances of ongoing growth, lending practices will likely tighten. Lending will become more conservative, as already appears to be happening. The collateral seemingly provided by the assumption of unending growth in the economy will probably diminish further each time fossil fuel shortages shock the economy.

This combination of inadequate supplies of fossil fuels to grow the economy and the probable reductions in lending money that previously supported growth will likely significantly undermine future growth in the world economy. The capitalist economic system may seem threatened, since growth operates as a fundamental driver of the economy.

Populations Increase as Fossil Fuels Decrease

The population explosion that has accompanied the increasing use of fossil fuels exacerbates the dangers involved. As populations increase exponentially on the global level (Daly, Martenson, Fitz-Gerald, and Moors, 2012), demand increases. In contrast, supplies of vital resources such as fossil fuels will eventually decrease. In this emerging world, supply and demand conflicts will increase over limited resources.

Yet we often lack adequate skills to manage such conflicts, especially in relation to our predispositions to compete and fight. Our capitalist economic system has historically thrived on competition and, thereby, reinforces us to compete for limited resources. This encourages competition rather than cooperation to solve such global problems—further exacerbating the danger of conflicts. For instance, competition for vital resources will likely elicit fear and reactivity based on our evolutionarily defaulted brain functions. When competition drives our behavior relative to limited global resources and fear initiates our reactive brain functions, we increasingly use our limited capacities, instead of the strengths of our higher cognitive brain functions, to create the future. Accordingly, we invite devolutionary consequences.

Devolution—Cultural Evolution Level

The successes of capitalism during the Industrial Age propelled this economic system into worldwide favor to lead us into the future. Unfortunately, the effectiveness of the economic system that developed during the industrial stage of our "Cultural" evolution appears destructive at times in our current Information Age and appears increasingly destructive for our future Age of Conscious Evolution (Hubbard, 2012).

An apparent assumption embedded in the capitalist system that seemed acceptable in past centuries held that people and planetary resources seemed essentially limitless. Meanwhile, the production of goods and services clearly seemed limited. Hence, the laws of supply and demand applied well to these limited supplies of goods and services. Monetary values could be ascribed to these specific products, while monetary values could not be easily ascribed to the apparent limitless supplies of people and planetary resources. In addition, people and the planet appeared too complex to define in monetary terms. In contrast to specific goods and services that seem to function as separate quantifiable entities, people and the planet function more through relationships and as whole systems. Thus, people and the environments of the planet that function in relationships and in interdependent oneness emerged as externalities in the capitalist system that more effectively values separate objects in material reality.

The Economic System Relies Ultimately on People and the Planet

Although the economic system has led to remarkable cultural progress, the capitalist system, like all economic systems, ultimately depends upon people and planetary resources for its existence. Without people and the planet, the economic system simply devolves. Meanwhile when breakdowns in human and planetary systems occur, the economic system can face realistic risks of devolution. For instance, disruptions to the workforce and consumers due to a global financial meltdown, a disease pandemic, or war-torn populations can threaten the health and sustainability of the economic system. Similarly, the lack of environmental resources—such as fossil fuels to power the economy, rare earth minerals to generate technological growth, the lack of water supplies from fresh water depletion, and the lack of food from soil erosion and changing weather patterns—constitute significant threats to the economic order.

As the great recession that started in December 2007 demonstrates, the global economic system operates in a complex interconnected network that must remain in balance and that when disrupted, can quickly spin out of control. Such disruptions can originate from internal imbalances within the system (such as the lack of regulations over special interest pursuits) or can be instigated by external human and environmental events (for example, wars or shortages of fossil fuels). The consequences of an economic meltdown today can affect not only local and national economies, but the entire global community with unknown consequences for the fate of humanity.

An Addiction to Fossil Fuels Exists

An addiction to fossil fuels seems prevalent across most human cultures at this time. In the current circumstances, an addiction refers to an attachment to an object or process that provides short-term pleasure (similarly, it can enable the temporary avoidance of negative experiences), but in the end it generates destruction. The addiction requires the development of a habit to repeat and perpetuate the benefits, until eventually enough damages accumulate, so devolution begins.

In the capitalist economic system addictions to money and consumption commonly arise. (Since the capitalist system depends upon continuing growth, addictions to money and consumption appear as important, maybe even as necessary processes that help the economy continue to grow.) Since fossil fuels supply most of the surplus physical energy that makes the economic system function, an addiction to fossil fuels almost naturally accompanies our economic success. Yet the addiction usually remains in the background beyond our normal awareness.

Presently, we require fossil fuels to remain available in order to perpetuate our past economic successes. Unfortunately, fossil fuels are finite and nonrenewable and lack sustainability themselves, as well as for the global economy. Since addictions tend to preclude people from awakening to and then initiating healthy responses to the situation, such as developing renewable fuels, we remain largely in denial. In addictions, short-term success often leads to long-term destruction and devolution. In this case, as peak oil approaches, demands will eventually outstrip supplies. The dominoes of our complex, fossil fuel dependent society will start to fall and potentially generate a crash in which we may "hit bottom." Of course, before this happens we have the capacity to awaken to our addiction and choose to grow and evolve to meet our needs in ways that align more appropriately with *reality*, as described in the following evolution section and in chapter 10.

Devolution—Human Evolution Level

As we cocreate to satisfy our short-term desires, we inadvertently contribute to the potential long-term devolution of the planet and our species. Consequently, "Human" evolution increasingly seems threatened. Ironically, these threats arise largely from our own actions. The limitations in our consciousness that trap us in self- and group-centered special interests restrict our perceptions of the evolutionary consequences of our actions.

Meanwhile, when we view these threats through the eyes of separateness, fears generally arise. These fears can automatically activate our amygdala into the fight, flight, and freeze reactivity that saved human lives from immediate physical danger during our early evolutionary history. Although most perceived death threats do not actually threaten our lives today, our reactive brains immediately apply old solutions to the current problem. These old solutions generally fail to solve current problems and sometimes spiral us into cycles of win-lose competition that can eventuate in violence that moves us toward devolution.

In contrast to Einstein's recommendation to solve problems by perceiving beyond the thinking that created the problem, we act with primitive survival reactions that apply solutions from our early personal, cultural, or even species history. Naturally, we fail to solve most present-day problems. In effect, amygdala reactivity devolves us internally as we react subconsciously with old solutions rather than respond consciously with our creative, higher cognitive capacities. Ultimately, this internal devolution in both our consciousness and our reactions can lead to external devolution in the world.

Devolution—Biological Evolution Level

The interdependent web of existence relies on the diversity of species and the complexity of ecosystems to maintain life on the planet. Human life exists within and depends upon this intricate web. Nevertheless, the progress of human culture that remains addicted to fossil fuels has often proceeded at the expense of strands within the web, as well as at the cost of interconnected portions of the web. For instance, many strands have been removed in recent years with the extinction of numerous plants and animals. Destruction and disruptions of ecosystems occur throughout the world, as rain forests disappear, desertification occurs, and fish populations shrink. The degradation of air, water, soils, and biological resources can impair our health, food security, consumer choices, and business opportunities (TEEB, 2009).

We frequently live from the perspective provided by the lens of separateness. From this isolated perspective we fail to appreciate the rich diversity of our interconnected, interdependent relationships. We do not notice our natural relationships with all the strands of the web, as well as with the web as a whole. Consequently, we naïvely exploit other participants and our relationships within this web, as we continue to undermine the biological integrity of the planet.

Devolution—Physical Evolution Level

The planet exists as a miniscule physical object in the spaciousness of the universe. From the evolutionary perspective, our lives depend on this finite collection of evolved stardust that represents "home" to all people. The air, land, and water that combine to form Earth provide essential but finite resources that enable us to live. Resources, such as fossil fuels, risk depletion as we burn them to produce energy for our immediate needs and desires. We simultaneously lose the greater value of oil, for instance, in the production of pharmaceutical drugs, plastics, and multiple other products that are derived from petroleum. As we burn these finite nonrenewable resources, our legacy to future generations goes up in smoke. Simultaneously, the pollution that results accelerates climate change and further denigrates our legacy.

Fossil fuels represent a hidden treasure buried for millions of years that embody ongoing value for the world. Yet we burn them for our short-term gain and, in the process, convert them into long-term costs for the world. When we fail to notice the consequences of our actions on the air, land, and water, we affect each of these planetary resources separately, as well as affect their interconnected relationships and the functioning of the whole planet.

On the local level when we combust fossil fuels to generate heat and energy, the by-products include carbon dioxide, ozone, nitrogen oxides, sulfur dioxide, heavy metals, and other pollutants. For instance, the disruption of the ozone layer in Earth's stratosphere threatens plants, marine ecosystems, and people with deadly radiation from space. Carbon dioxide emitted on local levels can accumulate on the global level to unbalance and change the climate. The devolutionary consequences of global climate change include more extreme, destructive storms, droughts, wildfires, and worldwide flooding from rising seas. Human consequences are less predictable due to our actions and reactions, but Professor James Lovelock, a top British climate scientist, warns that more than six billion people could die in this century due to changes in the climate (Polya, 2008).

Devolution—Spiritual Evolution Level

The ground of being ("God") provides the infinite potential from which evolutionary form arises. *Reality* embraces the whole as the oneness provided by the unity of the ground of being and evolutionary form. We perceive it most fully through our capacities for nondual awareness in which potential and form are inseparable as one (Wilber, 2004; 2006). Yet as separate human beings, we typically fail to notice our relationships, let alone our inherent oneness with *reality*. Our egocentric and ethnocentric perspectives portray ourselves as separate people at the center of the universe. We act like miniature gods with our personal perceptions and desires experienced as the truth. From these limited perspectives, we naturally fail to live in integrity with the increasingly larger truths of *reality*. As a result, we unknowingly exploit the relationships and oneness of the whole. In the process, we invite the devolution of ourselves, as well as the devolution of many other evolutionary creations. In the end, we fail to awaken to and develop our inherent spiritual, human being nature.

Evolution—Long-Term Benefits from Evolutionary Planning and Actions to Develop Health and Sustainability

Evolution—Self

Two Motivations for Conscious Evolution

Evolution often proceeds due to the threat of devolution (Hubbard, 2012). At this time we face enough devolutionary threats, including from fossil fuels, to motivate us to initiate evolutionary actions. Fortunately, we have the innate capacities to evolve, not only from fear regarding the consequences if we do not change, but also from our aspirations to grow and achieve higher purposes. In this latter case, we can employ our capacities for conscious evolution to grow intentionally to benefit ourselves and the world simultaneously. In other words, we evolve with fear to save or maintain our lives, while we evolve with hope to grow and enhance our lives. When we evolve motivated by aspirations to grow, we tend to experience greater freedom, happiness, love, and oneness in relationship to *reality*.

Evolution, when motivated by fear, provokes our brain to react in efforts to survive as the priority—survival living. Our higher cognitive functions for problem solving and planning diminish, as our older evolutionary brain functions react to save us. We automatically apply previously learned solutions to the present situation to maintain our existence. If these efforts prove unsuccessful, fear and desperation may provide us with the remote opportunity to awaken suddenly to an evolutionary growth solution.

In contrast to these rare, spontaneous insights generated from desperation, our brain has the cognitive capacities to explore and intentionally cocreate guided by the natural motivation to evolve. In such cases, proactive efforts enhance our chances to evolve. In addition, when we engage in conscious evolution we can create opportunities to transcend our normal limitations and the accompanying suffering associated with fear and survival living. Although both fear and growth motivated evolution can contribute to the success of our vision to create a healthy sustainable future, conscious evolution that integrates sustainability with healthy growth represents our best choice.

Two Types of Conscious Evolution

To complement the growth and fear motivations associated with evolution, two types of conscious evolution exist that can contribute to healthy sustainable living. The first involves our consciousness. It pertains to increases in our awareness of *reality*, as well as our commitment to live in integrity with the whole, as we pursue a conscious vision for healthy sustainable living. The second type of conscious evolution depends upon our actions. In this case, we need to evaluate both the short- and long-term consequences of our actions, especially in regard to evolutionary and devolutionary potential outcomes. We move toward our vision for health and sustainability when we integrate our consciousness and our actions so they perform congruently with the larger evolutionary processes. The prevention of harm and devolution in the world needs prioritized as we proceed.

Individually, we each have the capacity and the responsibility to cocreate in service to evolution and to all that supports our lives. The present opportunity to initiate conscious evolution for the benefit of all likely represents a first in human history, and potentially a last opportunity. We now have the capability to expand our awareness to perceive *reality* more fully than ever before. This consciousness opens the door to choose and act harmoniously for the benefit of ourselves, our relationships, and evolution as a whole.

Expand Consciousness into Worldcentric and Kosmocentric Perspectives

To step into this moment in history and capitalize on our potential to contribute to the beneficial transformation of ourselves, humanity, the planet, and evolution, we must continue to expand our consciousness into worldcentric and kosmocentic perspectives. These more inclusive perspectives encompass both personal egocentric and group ethnocentric viewpoints, while they expand our awareness into planetary and universal perspectives respectively. Ultimately, sustainability requires that our self, our groups, the world, and *reality* function in interdependent relationships that support a unified whole that necessitates that we perceive through our highest levels of consciousness.

The best way to expand our consciousness involves the practice of meditation (Wilbur, 2006). As we learn to let go of our normal attachments and conceptualizations of *reality*, we can access more of what exists and has the potential to exist in the universe. Another way to expand our consciousness involves following the natural processes of evolution. In this case, we can intentionally redirect our awareness from our separateness, and instead, focus on our relationships and natural oneness with all. We gain access to more of *reality* to integrate into our personal reality when we intentionally perceive our separateness, relationships, and oneness perspectives together as each reveals crucial processes of *reality*.

The Healthy Living Models Expand Consciousness and Actions to Harmonize Increasingly with Reality

The healthy living models provide further opportunities to expand our consciousness into worldcentric and kosmocentric perspectives of *reality*, so we can effectively pursue healthy sustainable living. These models overcome at least eight major perceptual limitations that restrict our consciousness that then undermine our ability to live in harmony with the world.

1. The models enable us to perceive more than our normal four to six items at one time. Thus, we can finally consciously perceive and work with the multiplicity of dimensions and levels in life that contribute to healthy sustainable living.

2. We can perceive a pictorial representation of each separate health dimension, its interactive relationships with other dimensions, and how they synergize to form a unified whole person. Thus, the models enable us to perceive through the separateness, relationship, and oneness lenses necessary to perceive *reality* more accurately and fully, so we can consciously integrate all aspects of our lives into healthy sustainable functioning.

3. The models enable us to perceive the internal complexity of our personal and collective lives and also perceive the external complexity of society and planetary existence. We can then synchronize our internal lives with the external world so we unify them into healthy sustainable lifestyles.

4. The models reveal our universal nature in which we quest for health and sustainability that generates a shared vision to unite humanity in service to higher purposes.

5. We experience the capacity to perceive multiple contributors to problems, instead of the few that we normally detect, so we can prioritize, synchronize, and act through a balanced approach of treatment, prevention, and wellness interventions to ameliorate previously unsolvable problems.

6. All dimensions and all levels ideally need to function in healthy manners to support individual health. Reciprocally, individuals, groups, and humanity need to function in healthy manners to support each other and all evolutionary processes, so we function together as an interdependent whole to promote health and sustainability.

7. The models synthesize into the ethical living model that enables us to forecast problems, especially devolutionary ones, so we finally have a basic universal system of ethics to guide us along the evolutionary path.

8. An integrated, healthy sustainable living model maximizes our abilities to engage in responsible conscious evolution with *reality* to cocreate a successful, sustainable future.

Evolution—Family

The family typically functions as the original source of information about how to define and interact with *reality*. Consequently, the consciousness level of the parents and other family members provides views of the world to the children consistent with egocentric, ethnocentric, worldcentric, or kosmocentric perspectives. A quest to expand the consciousness of parents to the worldcentric and kosmocentric levels has the potential to generate a multiplier effect in relation to their children. Parents can transmit more inclusive, accurate versions of *reality*, consistent with age-appropriate learning, to their children and to others involved in the family. This intentional teaching of information improves the opportunities for the children and others to grow into higher levels of consciousness. Parents have the responsibility to practice proactive consciousness and actions that contribute to an increasingly healthy sustainable world. In the process, they model and teach their children how to benefit themselves, humanity, and the world.

In regard to fossil fuels, the family represents a powerful influence regarding how to transition from the present priority of material consumption to the consumption of information and spiritual awakenings. In addition, the family can teach and model how to use the energy from fossil fuels efficiently. They can convey the ethic of conservation of finite, nonrenewable resources such as oil, coal, and natural gas. Such conservation efforts can benefit improved health due to decreases in pollution and at the same time can preserve fossil fuels for future generations to use in potentially more productive ways. The practice of recycling resources to maintain their functional integrity and the practice of conscious evolution to grow and maintain human life provide crucial gifts toward sustaining future generations.

The healthy, societal, and ethical living models help the family operate with expanded awareness and choices regarding *reality*. Progressively teaching children about how to realize health in the different dimensions of their lives, appropriate to their age, can prepare them to make healthy choices and balance the complexity of life. Teaching them that their personal health depends upon the health of all levels of society and the world invites them to participate in improving life for all people and species. As their brain develops, they can learn how different dimensions and different levels of society and the environment interrelate, so they can generate more beneficial outcomes. They can incorporate these models naturally into their lives, so they learn to include the major dimensions, their relationships, and their balance naturally into healthy sustainable lifestyles. In the process, children can learn how to contribute in increasingly ethical and evolutionary manners to others and the world.

Evolution—Business

We need to conserve fossil fuels as well as improve their efficient use in the workplace. From a different perspective, we need to learn to value and measure the human and planetary costs associated with their use. The capitalist economic system has traditionally relied upon the gross national product (GNP) as a primary measure of value to document economic progress. Nevertheless, GNP considers economic output and monetary income but fails to account for the natural wealth and assets upon which the economy depends. A new accounting of wealth needs to include manufactured capital (such as GNP), natural capital (for example, forests, wetlands, and air quality), and human and social capital (The World Bank, 2012a).

Wealth accounting provides an opportunity to assess whether growth is sustainable. For instance, when we include natural capital and human capital in economic decision making, we perceive *reality* more fully. As a result, we create choices in how we can evolve capitalism into better alignment with the world, so we can actively promote health and sustainability.

Since GNP focuses on money and material production, it omits much of *reality*. For instance, when a country uses its fossil fuels, it actually depletes its wealth. It grows its GNP in the short-term by exploiting its mineral assets, but endangers its long-term growth as it depletes these resources. It succeeds in capital production, while it diminishes its natural material wealth and pollutes both its human and natural wealth. Therefore, despite the appearance of an economy on an evolutionary path, GNP alone predisposes us to a devolutionary path.

Manufactured, Natural, and Human Capital Contribute to Sustainability

A sustainable path appears increasingly possible with the recent adoption by the UN Statistical Commission of the System for Environmental and Economic Accounts (SEEA). The SEEA provides an internationally agreed upon method to measure the wealth of natural material resources, such as fossil fuels, timber, and fisheries (The World Bank, 2012b). Countries around the world now need to learn how to utilize SEEA and employ it in decision making.

Human capital, similar to manufactured and natural capital, requires that we develop measurement tools. For instance, the healthy living model applied on the individual, family, business, community, and nation levels can indicate strengths and deficiencies in the different health dimensions on each level of society (see Bougsty, 2012 and chapter 8 for examples). In addition, the model can be used to identify imbalances among the dimensions as they attempt to function as a whole unit. With the aid of the comprehensive healthy living model, the results of these previous assessments can be translated into conscious evolution efforts to intervene systematically with treatment, prevention, and wellness interventions. These actions can coordinate on each level and across the levels to initiate systematic, transformative changes due to their standardized, comprehensive methodologies.

Another method to measure human capital involves calculating the costs of different human problems, such as described in chapter 5. For instance, the direct costs of treatment and the indirect costs in terms of lost productivity that result from mental health problems, alcohol and drug abuse, or physical diseases can be calculated. These costs can then be projected into the future based on the normal treatment expenses at expected prevalence rates. In comparison, projections can also be made for different prevention interventions relative to their costs and savings. Finally, projections for costs and savings associated with wellness interventions can be made, so we can systematically compare the treatment, prevention, and wellness alternatives. Combinations of wellness, prevention, and treatment interventions, in that order, will likely prove most effective.

An example of a wellness intervention involves teaching people how to improve their lives by using the healthy living model to assess, intervene, and monitor their lives, the health of their relationships, and the health of their family. Such direct interventions to improve health have the potential to avoid significant suffering in life and save tremendous amounts of money. Using the model longitudinally, we systematically establish personal goals and then evolve them to meet our developing needs. Like other conscious evolution processes, the more we set and pursue goals, and ideally, set missions or visions for our lives, the more likely we will evolve toward our goals and visions to improve healthy living.

The Evolution of the Capitalist Economy

The capitalist economic system needs to evolve in at least the following ways to prevent the devolutionary outcomes associated with the present system. Simultaneously, we need to evolve the capitalist system to support the growth and maintenance of a healthy sustainable future. In this section I offer the following suggestions:

- *Value*: Life is the greatest value for humanity. Health and sustainability exemplify vital components of our precious life. Consciousness functions at the core of our health and potentials for sustainable growth. Therefore, as our consciousness expands, we can act more responsibly so our health and sustainability can expand. In terms of our consciousness, we can prioritize how to perceive and evolve our multi-dimensional individual and collective capabilities, so we optimize our freedom, creativity, and happiness.

  Meanwhile, money presents a standardized, convenient measure of value for exchanging goods and services that can support and contribute to these more meaningful life goals. Money evolves from performing as the primary measure of value in the traditional capitalist economy to measuring value within exchanges that support the paramount value of healthy sustainable living.

  Wealth accounting replaces the gross national product as a measure of economic success. In this case, the combination of manufacturing capital, natural capital, and human capital integrate to measure value within the evolved economy that includes more of *reality*.

  The evolutionary ethical living model evaluates potential evolutionary and devolutionary outcomes. In addition, the model introduces a universal perspective of value that complements the wealth accounting methods. The combination of the ethical living model and wealth accounting introduces a more complete purpose for humanity—to create wealthy, healthy sustainable living. Consequently, our economy can now serve this higher purpose—to evolve humanity successfully and ethically into a wealthy, healthy sustainable future. This new comprehensive vision can guide the economy, and in turn, the economy can contribute to a future worthy of our greatest human potentials.

- *Process*: We need to learn to shift from our dependence on material reality and follow the inclusive processes of evolution to create a viable future. This means transforming our separateness through relationships to create more complex functioning for the benefit of all. Cooperative relationships need to develop to exchange unique forms of creativity to produce a more organized, orderly, fully functioning whole. When the producer, consumer, all humanity, the planet, and evolution win simultaneously in "win-win-win-win-win" fashion, then we advance the evolutionary process. This exemplifies love in action.

- *Goal*: Growth shifts progressively from material consumption that prioritizes meeting basic needs for survival and maintenance and shifts into information consumption and spiritual awakenings that fulfill the needs for conscious evolution. Spiritual awakenings reveal our deeper relationships and oneness with *reality*, so we gain the wisdom to utilize our informational knowledge more successfully on our evolutionary journey.

- *Motivation*: Successful evolution proceeds when we convert the competition among separate creative possibilities into cooperative creativity. We can then organize and order the relationships among the creations to form new wholes that perform beyond the sum of its separate parts.

  As cooperation and conscious evolution succeed, trust builds. Collective motivations can emerge between corporations, communities, nations, and the global community to create an increasingly sustainable future for all. In the process, we learn how to integrate our humanity and all levels of *reality* into a mutually functioning whole.

- *Rights*: Collective, public and planetary interests need to balance with private, special interests. When the two interests conflict, then the collective interests need to be prioritized, as they encompass more of *reality* and ultimately support the special interests.

- *Power*: The culmination of power in evolution involves integrating separate perspectives, relationships, and functioning as a whole. Thus, we need to shift our early evolutionary tendencies for power through authoritarian, self-interests and instead grow based on developing our capabilities for participatory democratic processes that value and include all perspectives.

Healthy and Ethical Living Models to Evolve Businesses

To improve the functioning of our businesses and corporations, so they contribute to the vision for healthy sustainable living, we can employ the healthy and ethical living models. For instance, we can use the healthy living model to improve functioning within the business to measure how well it contributes to healthy living for employees, consumers, and the broader society. The ethical living model can then help identify how well the goods and services produced contribute to humanity and the planet, and even more importantly, what devolutionary risks they pose.

In these ways, the business community can employ tools that align their work and productivity with the universal vision for healthy sustainable living. These tools expand our perceptions of *reality*, so the American Dream for success can evolve into the more comprehensive Universal Dream for Healthy Sustainable Living. Accordingly, we integrate our efforts to generate an evolutionary path into the future.

Evolution—Community

The community setting offers the opportunity to evolve from our inherent separateness into our natural relationships with others. When we consciously evolve from perceptions of living separately with a collective of people and instead perceive living in relationship with the community as an extension of ourselves, we transform the experience of community. In the process, we awaken to our responsibilities to care for all the participants and the collective environment and ultimately serve all in healthy manners.

From this collective viewpoint, we can develop cooperative neighborhoods, organizations, and businesses. These cooperative ventures can help us transcend our competitive habits and evolve into working together. We shift into functioning as a collective in which all realities count and contribute to increased opportunities to organize at a higher degree of order. We can evolve personally and collectively in alignment with evolution that transports us naturally from competitive separateness into cooperative relationships. The creativity that arises in cooperative relationships can generate increased organization, order, and oneness. This evolutionary process can be especially cultivated when a group meditates together to awaken to higher levels of consciousness and collective realizations (Cohen, 2012; Hamilton, 2012b; Hubbard, 2012; Patten, 2012). In these ways we increasingly align with evolution as we advance our functioning into more complex, orderly living. When we work together, create, and agree on new ways to achieve success, we follow the path of evolution in which we awaken to greater unity and oneness than previously available.

More specifically, we can work to conserve fossil fuels as well as contribute to healthy living by developing economic cooperatives. These cooperatives can share work and resources to benefit the participants and the community as a whole. Such cooperative efforts advance evolutionary processes from traditional, win-lose competition among separate players to win-win cooperation among community members. Democratic communications and employee ownership of businesses in the community can further enhance this cooperative spirit (see chapter 6). Communities can also develop collective living settings in which residents share material resources, exchange information, and work to form healthy, cooperative relationships.

We can intentionally work to establish sustainable communities through consciously planning for that end. Examples of issues to consider include transportation, heating and cooling, housing, and manufacturing that increasingly utilizes nonpolluting, renewable energy sources. Local production of food, energy, and consumer goods and services can minimize pollution that stimulates devolutionary processes. Improvements in human capital can occur by creating opportunities for people to participate cooperatively with deep listening, democratic decision making, planning, dispute resolution, mediation, and collective meditation.

We can further support community growth with the help of our societal institutions. We can transform our education system, the media, health care, and the democratic political systems to teach and model functioning at higher levels of consciousness that benefit the community (see chapter 6). Each institution can support people to develop increasingly accurate, inclusive views of *reality*. As we perceive more precisely, we can individually and collectively choose evolutionary rather than devolutionary actions and lifestyles.

Healthy, Societal, and Ethical Living Models Applied to the Community

A method is needed to help integrate all these concerns so they coordinate and synergize harmoniously in service to the larger vision for healthy sustainable living. The healthy, societal, comprehensive, and ethical living models can facilitate this process. Individuals can improve their personal health through use of the healthy living model (see Bougsty, 2012). Individuals, families, organizations, businesses, and the community can use the societal and comprehensive models to integrate and improve healthy functioning across all levels of the community. The ethical living model can help the community assess if any actions on any levels of society contribute to devolutionary risks. Such risks need stopped, modified, or replaced using appropriate positive alternatives to support sustainable outcomes.

Evolution—Nation

With increasing signs of devolutionary outcomes, the nation needs to develop sustainable energy policies. This means shifting priorities from fossil fuel use to renewable, nonpolluting sources of energy. Along these lines, subsidies need to shift from fossil fuels to instead support innovation and the development of alternative fuels that avoid devolutionary consequences. We need to create a blueprint that guides the development and use of energy resources. The short- and long-term interests of the population and the consequences for people and the environment need to be integrated and balanced in order to support a healthy sustainable future.

Societal, Comprehensive, and Ethical Living Models Help Evolve the Nation

The societal and comprehensive healthy living models provide the means to transform a nation to develop healthy living throughout the population (see chapter 8). Treatment interventions for problems experienced across different levels of society can reduce the devolutionary pull they exert on the rest of society. Prevention interventions can protect the maintenance of the nation, whenever devolutionary threats arise. Finally, wellness interventions can proactively stimulate the growth necessary to evolve the nation further into healthy living. These interventions can be integrated and prioritized to synergize successful changes across all the health dimensions and levels of society. In these ways, the nation can effectively and comprehensively transform into healthy living. The ethical living model complements these changes by assuring that the transformation leads to long-term sustainable living.

Evolution—World

The finite nature of fossil fuels, particularly peak oil with its enormous devolutionary potentials, challenges the global community to shift from competition into worldwide cooperation. The global pollution generated by fossil fuels further challenges us to work together as a world community. We need to learn to communicate, cooperate, and develop plans for the collective benefit of the world's population and the planetary environment. In these processes, we naturally encourage the expansion of consciousness into the worldcentric and kosmocentric levels.

In an effort to confront the finite nature of fossil fuels, we need to prioritize the development of nonpolluting, renewable energy alternatives. To facilitate this shift, we can phase out global subsidies for fossil fuels, estimated to be $775 billion in 2012 and redirect these financial aides into alternative fuels. These fossil fuel subsidies amount to twelve times the amount provided in support of renewable energies. If fossil fuels subsidies are phased out by 2020, a nearly 6 percent reduction in carbon dioxide emissions can be expected (NRDC, 2012). As a complement to these alternative energies, we also need to stabilize the global population, so the demand for energy, as well as other finite resources, can balance with the supply.

Essentially, we need to develop a movement designed to create a viable future for humanity. The universal motivations for health and sustainability make the vision for healthy sustainable living a natural choice for a global movement. We will need to organize and apply the healthy living models on the local to the global levels to realize this vision. Along these lines, healthy living can be systematically developed among individuals throughout the world (see Bougsty, 2012), as well as among their families, communities, businesses, nations, and as a global community. With the societal and comprehensive models we can address the complexity of survival, maintenance, and growth issues throughout all dimensions of life and levels of the world. Ultimately, the ethical living model provides the necessary overview to guide our choices on how to create sustainable, healthy living for humanity.

Evolution—Cultural Level

The Evolution of Our Capitalist Economic System

The capitalist economic system has greatly accelerated cultural progress. The successes of the system excelled during the Industrial Age. Nevertheless, the economy must evolve in order to meet the changing needs in the Information Age and, especially, the emerging Age of Conscious Evolution. In particular, the capitalist economy needs to evolve to value human and planetary costs and benefits as inherent parts of the system rather than considering them as externalities. People and the planet actually serve as the core ingredients of the economic system. For example, without people and the planet, the economic system would simply not exist. Meanwhile, when breakdowns in human and planetary systems do occur, devolutionary threats to the economy can result. Since the economy depends upon both people and the environment for its survival and sustenance, the system has to evolve to value and hold both as essential components for its future existence.

The past successes of the capitalist economy have depended significantly upon people and the planet being considered as externalities. Under this value system, the special private interests that largely drive our economy can compete and in the process exploit the planet, as witnessed by disruptions in ecosystems, extinction of species, and global climate change. This special interest focus also neglects and can exploit people, thereby contributing to a world of haves and have-nots. For instance, in 2006, 497 billionaires had twice the monetary worth of 2,400,000,000 people in poor countries. Furthermore, nearly half the people in the world experience problems of inadequate water supplies and basic sanitation necessary for healthy lives (Global Issues, 2010).

Nevertheless, universal human services (including education, water, sanitation, nutrition, and reproductive and health services) could be delivered to people in developing countries for an estimated additional forty billion dollars. Unfortunately, other values dominate in the world driven largely by special interests. For instance, military spending costs nearly twenty times what is needed to provide these universal human services (Human Development Reports, 2011). In combination, the lack of clean water, sanitation, and adequate food leads to suffering and dying in impoverished conditions, as well as to increasing threats of violence and terrorism around the world.

The future of the economic system needs to shift to prioritize human and planetary concerns. For instance, when a conflict occurs in which devolutionary harm to people and the planet may occur, the protection of humanity and Earth needs to be prioritized. The traditional production of goods and services that creates profits for special interests cannot be prioritized when immediate threats to human life exist. These private interests will continue to drive growth in the economy, but we can no longer risk growth that introduces devolutionary threats to our future. In other words, the economy must evolve to protect collective human and planetary interests that keep us all alive as more fundamental and important than traditional private special interests, when the two conflict.

To assist in this process, the ethical living model can be used to identify potential costs and benefits of our actions across all levels of humanity and the planet. Such evaluations appear essential in order to prevent devolutionary outcomes. In addition, the ethical living model provides guidance on how to best support all the levels of *reality* and their interdependent relationships. It introduces a necessary tool for global ethics to support our quest to achieve the universal vision for healthy sustainable living.

Evolution—Human Level

Four critical ways to evolve humanity will be proposed in the following section. These proposals summarize previous discussions:

1. **Healthy sustainable living requires that our perceptions and actions function in harmony with *reality*.** The most fundamental threat to our future involves our limited perceptions of *reality*. When we perceive through the lens of separation, for instance, we perceive and act relative to our self and group interests. We fail to recognize the needs of the rest of the world; hence, we lack the awareness necessary to act in integrity with it all. Along these lines, we must work to increase our consciousness from unsustainable, egocentric and ethnocentric viewpoints to sustainable, worldcentric and kosmocentric perspectives. As we perceive more inclusive and accurate views of *reality* as a whole, we enhance our opportunities to create consciously and evaluate the potential impacts of our actions. To produce a vital future, we have to evolve our consciousness toward understanding the world as fully and accurately as possible, so we can act in coherence with all that supports our life.

2. **Conscious evolution needs to mirror the processes of evolution.** In general, conscious evolution proceeds through a sequence of steps. We need to function consistent with how evolution works, if we expect to participate in sustainable ways with the evolving world. Initially, the consciousness of a separate individual or collective of people generates unique creativity that leads to competition within the natural selection processes. Nevertheless, for evolution to proceed, relationships need to transition into cooperation, so the creation can undergo organization and develop sufficient order to integrate into oneness with the whole. The new, more complex whole further contributes to the evolution of the world.

   Presently, competition dominates our creative processes, as it aligns with the functioning of our capitalist economic system. Competition defines our relationships as separate individuals or groups against each other. Such perceptions of separateness often impair our health, but more fundamentally can undermine our sustainability. Nevertheless, separateness can also join in cooperative relationships, such as in the exchange of money for goods and services. Both producers and consumers appear to win in relation to their special interest sharing. While this economic cooperation may prove evolutionary in the short-term for the special interests of the parties, their limited views of *reality* may stimulate devolutionary consequences for people and the planet outside of their circle of interests. When such external devolution occurs, it can then undermine and devolve the success, and even the lives, of those pursuing the special interests.

To overcome this limited version of cooperation, we need to convert our perceptions and choices of actions, so they cooperate with the whole, as indicated by the ethical living model. When we cooperate and understand our different perceptions, we can organize and order our differences into more complex representations of *reality*. We can mutually create innovations, agreements, and actions that perform at higher levels. As we cooperate to increase our creativity and productivity, we also evaluate how to prevent harm to any aspects of *reality*. This balance between creative innovation and the protection from unforeseen harm enables us to evolve progressively toward healthy sustainable living.

3. **We need to evolve the reactive, devolutionary predispositions of our amygdala.** Artifacts from our evolutionary brain now threaten the future of humanity. In particular, the ancient brain functions of the amygdala react to save our life, but in modern times its fight, flight, and freeze reactions more likely endanger rather than save our lives. For instance, the amygdala automatically reacts to anything that appears to threaten our lives. Since our more advanced cortical brain functions have worked to solve most imminent threats to our physical life, the amygdala perceives almost exclusively imaginary death threats and reacts to them as real threats. These overreactions to imaginary threats are bad enough, but the amygdala now has modern weapons created by the higher brain with which to react. Weapons of mass destruction, operated under the control of our reptilian-like brain, place the future of humanity in jeopardy.

These primitive reactive processes can endanger our personal health, as well as endanger other people, the society, and global health. When we react in fear for our lives, the amygdala of the people around us can then feel threatened. A vicious cycle of reactivity can spiral us into devolutionary outcomes. Since our reactivity can now extend beyond the original reach of our hands and feet, and instead can extend anywhere in the world with bombs and biochemical weapons, we have to learn to retrain our amygdala to not react to imaginary threats.

We need to evolve consciously in order to overcome this evolutionary predisposition of our amygdala to react primitively to imaginary death threats. This reactive predisposition appears as a fundamental contributor to most of the violence in the world. We can utilize a variety of methods to expand our consciousness, so we can relax the vigilance and reprogram its reactivity. Examples of methods to retrain and evolve our amygdala include: meditation, hypnosis, energy work such as tapping on acupressure points (Ortner, 2012), HeartMath techniques to develop greater heart, brain coherence (Childre, Lew, Martin, and Beech, 2000), psychotherapy, and systematic desensitization to change reactive tendencies in a progressive manner.

4. **The healthy sustainable living models increase our perceptions and choices with** *reality*. Our evolutionary brain lacks the direct conscious capacities to perceive and interpret how to create healthy living, let alone how to create sustainable living. Therefore, we have to employ models to serve like pictures of a thousand words to coalesce multiple components into one interactive whole. These models portray crucial components of the world, their interactive relationships, and their ultimate functioning as a whole in one

inclusive picture. This comprehensive view of *reality* can help us consider all the major components and their relationships that contribute to the realization of the vision for healthy sustainable living that can help transport us into a viable future for humanity.

This fourth recommendation involves the need to perceive *reality* beyond the normal limitations of our sense organs and brain. The healthy, societal, comprehensive, and ethical living models are designed to help us perceive the complexity of *reality* that our evolutionary brain lacks the capabilities to perceive directly. In other words, each model provides progressively more inclusive maps of the whole that incorporates the separate pieces, their interdependent relationships, and their functioning as a whole that our brain cannot perceive without such aides. These models combine to help us systematically create healthy living for individuals, businesses, societies, and the world as a whole. The ethical living model enables us to evaluate and make certain that the special interest levels of healthy living do not significantly harm the rest of the web of life and *reality*. Healthy living that prevents unforeseen harm can then transcend us into sustainable living.

Consequently, such models provide necessary tools for conscious evolution. These tools contribute to human evolution as well in that we expand our perceptions and participation with *reality*. These models enable us to perceive beyond the limits of our sense organs that have carried us through most of our evolution. Nevertheless, our cortical brain has evolved our modern cultural innovations by perceiving increasingly into the world of information beyond our simple sensory perceptions. Thus, we evolve our personal and collective realities through our expanded awareness of information that we usually access by the objective methods of science.

As we perceive portions of *reality* more fully and accurately, we can develop new technologies that would not appear on the evolutionary scene through simple random mutations. These technologies that emerge from our evolution of information within our consciousness can actually change the material world in ways previously not available to humans. On the surface these changes usually appear evolutionary. Beneath the surface, however, we discover many devolutionary changes that also occur, but happen beyond our still limited perceptions of *reality*.

Therefore, we have to develop models like the healthy sustainable living models to expand our consciousness beyond our limited sense organs and the natural limitations in our evolutionary brain functions. Through such models we can appreciate and take responsibility for both the evolutionary and the devolutionary consequences of our modern-day actions. In doing so, we advance human evolution to cocreate and coexist with all other forms of evolution. In this way, healthy sustainable living becomes a more attainable goal for humanity.

Evolution—Biological Level

Evolution requires diversity among species and ecosystems in order to expand the potentials for transformation into higher levels of functioning. Any lack of diversity undermines the creative potential important to drive the system toward successful evolution. As inevitable changes occur, diversity also provides a safety net to increase the potential adaptability available to adjust to new circumstances and risks. We need to protect all species from extinction and ecosystems from destruction, as they provide the basic web of interconnected relationships that maintains our lives.

Furthermore, we can consider the potential economic expenses associated with prevention efforts that attempt to maintain functioning in comparison to treatment interventions that rehabilitate species and ecosystems. The example of climate change suggests that investments of 1 percent of global gross domestic product directed to prevent future damages may save an estimated 5 to 20 percent of global gross domestic product needed to confront the expected damages (Stern, 2006). In other words, the protection of species and ecosystems will naturally be much more economical and effective than attempting to repair damages to nature.

In addition, our treatment interventions to repair damages to ecosystems, for example, may appear like inserting a thread or two into a tapestry of the web of life that has evolved throughout evolutionary history. The complexity of the web and the multitude of cooperative relationships necessary for all the components to function must make our interventions seem like uninformed, competitive mutations. Most mutations probably die off in their unsuccessful competitive struggles with the established web and simply recycle back into the larger whole. Nevertheless, human mutations are not fully random as they derive from our awareness of portions of the web. They may fit into the web enough that their intended evolutionary changes may occur or at least partially develop. Devolutionary changes may also result however.

We need to prioritize the protection rather than the remediation of damages that occur to species and ecosystems. These species and ecosystems represent parts of the web that may be necessary for our survival. In addition, they carry the evolutionary heritage that successfully integrates competition and cooperation into viable relationships that generate life. We need to learn from this evolutionary heritage, so we can shift from our cultural heritage that focuses on competition. We need to advance our traditions of competition into the cooperation necessary for successful evolution. Healthy sustainable living depends upon the integration of our competition side into cooperation with all of *reality*.

Evolution—Physical Level

Physical evolution originally created the planet from stardust. The different elements that make up Earth exist in finite quantities; therefore, we live in a world of limited material resources. Consequently, our cocreative potentials in the material realm of *reality* are restricted as we do not create these elemental resources; nonetheless, we have to live within their finite limits. When we fail to recognize or respect the limited nature of these resources, our perceptions conflict with *reality*. Although we may desire more gold, silver, and fossil fuels, evolution, not humans, produced these resources. When our desires and actions fail to match *reality*, we step onto a devolutionary path.

Since our abilities to make these resources are limited, we have to expend increasing energy to seek and mine their remaining deposits. In the process, we usually further damage the land, water, and air resources that support our lives. Our perception of needs and the design of the economy to meet these needs usually gain our attention in the foreground. Meanwhile, the damage inflicted by our actions on the planetary environment usually remains in the background. As a result, we normally place our short-term needs and desires over the long-term damage that we initiate in regard to the global climate, oceans, and the ecosystems upon which our lives depend.

We now have the capacity to evaluate possible damages that may result from our actions by using the ethical living model. This comprehensive model enables us to evaluate damages from the local to the global levels in relation to both human and environmental concerns. Nevertheless, many of these threats to our lives can simply be avoided if we respect the finite limits of Earth's physical resources. We will eventually face limitations with all the fossil fuels similar to the approaching of peak oil. These fossil fuels are both finite and essentially nonrenewable.

With this in mind, we need our personal and collective realities to value the world and all *reality* that governs our evolution. This means that we learn to live within the limits of the physical resources present on Earth. Although we may have infinite potentials to cocreate with information and spiritual awakenings in our consciousness, in the material world we live with finite limits. We have to learn to respect the limitations of our cocreative abilities at this time relative to these finite material resources.

Evolution—Spiritual

Spiritual evolution from a personal standpoint depends on our perceptions of *reality*. Ultimately, spirit consists of all the potential of the ground of being and all manifestations of form in evolution that unify as *reality*. When we expand our consciousness, we increase our perceptions of *reality*, and thereby, we may experience spiritual awakenings. Such spiritual awakenings occur anytime we embody more of *reality*. Profound spiritual awakenings involve the realization that we connect as one with everything that simultaneously exist as separate forms, in interconnected relationships, and function in larger unified wholes as manifestations of infinite empty potential. This coexistence of separateness, relationships, and oneness permeates evolution and arises from the unmanifest potential of all. In this context, spiritual evolution occurs whenever we consciously experience more of *reality* than we previously perceived or when we change *reality* as a result of our consciousness and actions. Therefore, any awareness beyond what we presently know or conceptualize accesses spirit in new ways, and therefore, generates at least miniature spiritual awakenings.

As we perceive more of *reality*, we increase our capacities for survival. We increase our choices on how to protect, and conversely, how to grow in our mortal life. As we expand our perceptions of the world, we can see beyond our separateness, so we can consciously connect in our relationships. As we share information, energy, and material objects in our relationships, we make contributions to our immortal existence. As other people and the world are affected by our consciousness and behaviors, they perceive and transfer the information and material changes that we share into their personal reality. In this process, parts of our behaviors and consciousness are incorporated into others, who then pass these parts or modified portions onto others and the world. Accordingly, our mortal self evolves into others and evolutionary processes to generate our immortal existence.

Finally, whenever we experience the present moment as simple awareness of infinite empty potential, we realize our eternal nature. We awaken and expand our limited intelligence as we access portions of the universal intelligence embedded in all energy, information, and matter. Then when we awaken to both the empty potential of all associated with the ground of being and all manifest form in evolution, we can realize our integrated mortal, immortal, and eternal natures simultaneously in nondual consciousness

As an example, when we perceive from our normal sense of separateness, we can appreciate the relationships that connect us with the world, and in the process, we can sometimes experience a realization of oneness with all in our perceptual field. If we expand consciousness enough, we may experience or conceptualize the whole of *reality*—the Source and the Creation of all—that people sometimes call "God." When we increasingly perceive this whole, we can act in greater harmony with all. From this perspective, we can consciously become cocreators with God or the whole of *reality*.

The vision to create healthy sustainable living becomes increasingly viable from a personal, a species, a planetary, an evolutionary, and a spiritual perspective. We contribute to this vision when we cocreate innovations that simultaneously provide benefits, with no significant devolutionary consequences to us, the world, and all *reality*. In these ways, we function and cocreate as if we are "God's helpers." We contribute to the continuing creative evolution of the world. In these processes, we transform increasingly from our human nature into our spiritual nature. We progressively awaken to more of *reality*, so we integrate and act from our deepest human and spiritual natures—we evolve as spiritual human beings.

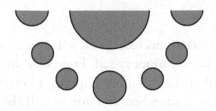

CHAPTER 10

Conscious Evolution Cocreates a Healthy Sustainable Future

● ● ● ● ● ● ●

In this final chapter, I will provide an overview of how to integrate the models and concepts presented in this book. Four major models work in concert to propel us toward our ultimate vision to create healthy sustainable living for all. A seven-step methodology supports these models, ranging from our innate impulse to evolve to our monitoring of the consequences of our actions. Conscious evolution toward a goal or vision, while operating from our highest stage of consciousness, enables us to select actions that we introduce consistent with the natural processes of evolution. We can then align our lives to function in increasing coherence with *reality*.

To create a viable future for humanity, we need to practice stewardship for other people and the planet. As other people and the environment enjoy health, they tend to support our health and happiness as well. Thus, we are challenged to transcend our customary approaches to growth that attempt to meet our basic comforts and satisfy our personal special interests. Our personal and group desires will continue, as they integrate into higher purposes intended to serve humanity, the planet, and evolution. Fortunately, these investments in the health of the rest of *reality* tend to increase the likelihood that benefits will return to us. These higher purposes challenge us to grow at the cutting edge of human consciousness, as well as at the cutting edge of evolution.

Amazingly, we appear to be the first species on Earth to confront the fact that the life of our species, as well as many others, rest in our hands. In a sense, we serve like miniature gods. To embrace this challenge, we need to awaken our innate capacity to expand our consciousness to prepare for this journey. We enjoy unique powers of awareness and brain functioning that allow us to perceive increasing views of *reality*. With more full and accurate perspectives of the *reality*, we have the capacities to choose and initiate actions that align productively with the world. Thus, we can cocreate evolutionary change that benefits the health and sustainability of ourselves and the world simultaneously.

To expand our consciousness, we first need to shift our awareness from the lens of separateness, which concludes that only our separate self and our accompanying special interests can create success. Instead, we need to perceive increasingly through the lens of relationships, so we act on behalf of the web of interdependent relationships that keeps us alive as a separate self. Through these two lenses we exist as an interconnected, social self, as well as a separate self. We also exist as a participant in evolution as an evolutionary self. From this universal perspective, we have the natural urge to evolve and contribute to evolution. Our evolutionary self exists in oneness with the universe and naturally acts to benefit the whole (Hamilton, 2012b). In the process, we create long-term benefits for our separate self and social self, whenever we act from our evolutionary self.

The Evolutionary Impulse Enlivens Us to Cocreate through Conscious Evolution

An "Evolutionary Impulse" to evolve exists at the core of evolution (Cohen, 2012; Hamilton, 2012b; see Figure 18). This impulse that drives all evolution functions in humans through four fundamental dynamics. These dynamics include our "Power," "Unique," "Worth," and "Love" that operate at the core of our evolutionary lives. These dynamics, however, exist beyond our normal perceptions. We need to expand our consciousness to experience these gifts. They empower us to perceive and act consistent with our ultimate nature as spiritual human beings. As a result, we cocreate in evolution through these dynamics that arise from the infinite potential of the ground of being.

Power—The first dynamic associated with the evolutionary impulse to evolve arose with the Big Bang (Hamilton, 2010) and energizes all evolutionary form with the power to evolve. As humans, we enjoy at least five basic means to participate with our power and fulfill our urge to evolve and, in the process, contribute to the processes of evolution:

1. *Consciousness*—simply being aware with no conceptualizations and no sense of a personal self provides the freedom to just be with the infinite potential of the ground of being. When we open our awareness to include evolutionary form as well as the empty potential of all, we experience nondual consciousness or the oneness of all *reality*.

2. *Personal Consciousness*—we conceptualize what our sense organs detect and our brain functions interpret from *reality*, so we can develop a limited, unique personal reality that we frequently think reveals the "truth" about *reality*.

3. *Conscious Choices* can emerge regarding how to act in the world relative to our personal reality.

4. *Actions* can follow our choices, and as a result, these behaviors introduce mutations into the world that can change *reality*.

5. *Conscious Cocreation*—represents our capacity to perceive *reality*, as fully and accurately as possible, so we can envision and choose how to participate in integrity with the world, so evolution and ourselves maintain or grow into improved health and sustainability.

Unique—The second dynamic of the evolutionary impulse involves unique contributions to evolution that contribute diversity for the natural selection processes. We introduce unique consciousness and unique actions that generate potential mutations into the competitive arena of natural selection. These unique forms of information and matter compete with other unique forms to produce the diversity important to maximize the potential for viable evolutionary changes.

Figure 18:
Conscious Processes that Contribute to Conscious Evolution

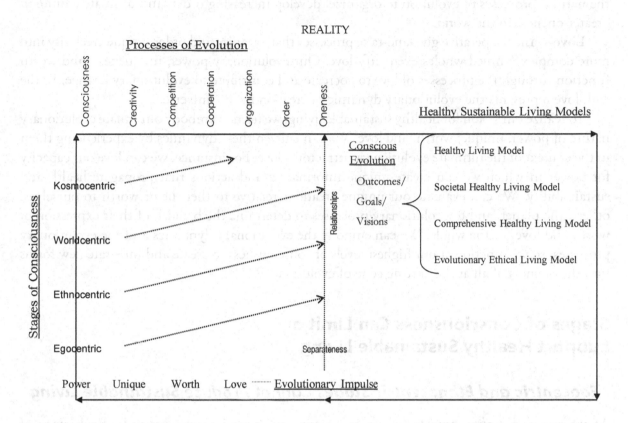

Worth—While our unique consciousness and actions have worth as they contribute to the natural selection processes, our worth increases as we move beyond competition and create through cooperation. The mutations that we introduce add increasing worth as we cooperate in the natural processes of evolution to organize, develop increasing order, and ultimately unite in greater oneness in the world.

Love—The cooperative give-and-take processes that organize and order unique creativity into more complex, unified wholes exemplify love. Our evolutionary power, uniqueness, and worth function through the processes of love to cocreate and contribute to evolutionary change. In the end, love represents the evolutionary dynamic of creation in the universe.

To realize our vision for healthy sustainable living, we need to embody our innate evolutionary nature of power, unique, worth, and love. We can enliven these dynamics by experiencing them in the context of the ultimate evolutionary attractor—love. For instance, we can love our capacity for power in which we can create unique information and actions that propagate health and sustainability. We can evaluate our unique creations relative to their fit or worth to ourselves, others, the planet, and to evolutionary processes to determine the breadth of their expression of worth and love for the whole. We can embody the evolutionary dynamics and the evolutionary processes, so we function at our highest levels of consciousness to create and integrate new forms into the oneness of all at the cutting edge of evolution.

Stages of Consciousness Can Limit or Support Healthy Sustainable Living

Egocentric and Ethnocentric Stages Cannot Produce Sustainable Living

As we perceive *reality* more fully and accurately, our consciousness expands. Each stage of consciousness perceives significantly more of the world. Initially, we perceive the world from an "Egocentric" perspective in which we appear as a separate self at the center of the universe (see Figure 18). As a result, we act in self-centered, special interest ways. When we expand our consciousness to include other people, an "Ethnocentric" perspective develops in which our identity group now appears at the center of the world. In this case, we act in group-centered, special interest ways (for instance, behaving for our family, organization, business, community, or nation). Although perceiving through the lens of relationships, the lens of separateness persists and still perceives us as a separate group within the world.

Both the egocentric and ethnocentric perspectives are necessary and valuable, but our consciousness from these two levels limits us to self- and group-centered perspectives. Therefore, the lack of a perspective of the whole world, upon which our lives depend, means that egocentric and ethnocentric perspectives can unknowingly harm people and the planet beyond our awareness. Hence, these perspectives are insufficient to create a healthy sustainable future for humanity and the planet.

A Worldcentric Perspective Is the Minimum Consciousness for Sustainability

Since 70 percent of the world's population functions at the egocentric and ethnocentric levels (Wilbur, 2006), we face a potential death threat for humanity, if we fail to expand enough people's consciousness into the "Worldcentric" perspective. From this global perspective, we begin to recognize and identify with all humanity and the planet. We perceive enough of *reality* to realize that our personal and group survival depends upon the survival of humanity and the planetary environments. Our circles of concern and self-interests expand to include the entire world. This inclusive consciousness introduces the potential to create healthy sustainable living more consistently, as our self, our groups, and the entire planet all simultaneously have value.

A Kosmocentric Perspective Introduces Consciousness for a Sustainable Future

The "Kosmocentric" perspective provides our best hope for the future. Ken Wilber (2010) estimates the tipping point to shift into a sustainable future requires ten percent of the population functioning at the integral stage of consciousness. This stage encompasses the worldcentric perspective and can expand into the kosmocentric perspective as well. From these perspectives, we progressively appreciate evolutionary form on the world level that can expand into the universe, and sometimes, even includes experiences with the infinite empty potential of the ground of being. As we perceive *reality* more fully, we substantially enhance our abilities to create healthy sustainable living. Furthermore, we can embrace our responsibilities to contribute to all—including our self, our group, the world, evolution, and all *reality*.

Conscious Evolution Follows the Processes of Evolution

We consciously cocreate with *reality* when we follow the "Processes of Evolution" (see Figure 18; also figures 1–3). In conscious evolution, we proceed through the processes in the following manner. Our personal consciousness stimulates a unique form of creativity that confronts competition with other unique or already established forms of consciousness and actions. Eventually, cooperation must replace competition to initiate the organization necessary to generate a higher order of complexity and oneness into the world.

Naturally, the processes of evolution emerge from and correspond with the dynamics of the evolutionary impulse. For instance, our consciousness derives from the *power* that enlivens our awareness, as well as activates our sensory and brain functions to create a *unique* personal reality. Our unique creations compete for *worth* in the broader world until the give-and-take exchange processes initiate the cooperation, organization, and order to create a more complex oneness that manifests via the dynamic of *love*.

The evolutionary impulse and the processes of evolution combine to help transform the "Separateness" of individual forms to interconnect through "Relationships" to create an interdependent unity of "Oneness." Thus, more complex wholes form in evolution. The sustainability of these new creations, however, depends significantly upon the level or stage of consciousness employed in their formation. For instance, the more expansive and inclusive our consciousness, the more potential we have to create complex new forms that integrate successfully with *reality*.

As we gain greater awareness, we can reduce the risks of devolutionary consequences as we consider potential harm before it occurs. Since egocentric and ethnocentric perspectives provide very limited versions of *reality* and simultaneously serve only self- or group-centered interests, operations from these levels of consciousness often inadvertently initiate destructive, devolutionary results. An example involves our use of fossil fuels that serve our special interests, but simultaneously generate devolutionary consequences for the global climate. In contrast, worldcentric perspectives reduce the risks of such accidental devolution on the planetary level, while kosmocentric perspectives provide the most promising path to protect ourselves from devolution, as we engage in conscious evolution relative to *reality* as a whole.

Evolution from Accidental Outcomes, Intentional Goals, and Collective Visions

Traditionally, evolution has proceeded by random mutations that generate accidental "Outcomes" (Figure 18). Notwithstanding, people contribute to accidental outcomes as well. For instance, when we act out impulsively, we may generate random changes. Furthermore, we may perform maintenance habits in subconscious fashions (for example, we automatically leave the lights on, accelerate our vehicle too rapidly, or eat without conscious awareness). In these ways, we can unintentionally, and seemingly randomly, harm other aspects of the world.

We change evolution in another manner when we consciously set "Goals" and initiate actions on their behalf. In the process of attaining a goal, we can be most effective by following the processes of evolution that naturally generate change. For instance, we create a goal that may compete with other possible goals, until we decide to cooperate, organize, and order our lives to achieve this new, more complex way of functioning. We further expand our evolutionary potential when we participate in the creation and pursuit of collective goals. In this case, we engage in relationships with other individuals and then cooperate and organize, order, and realize the goal. We sometimes achieve outcomes that previously seemed impossible.

We substantially expand our evolutionary potentials when we personally and then collectively create long-term "Visions" for our conscious evolution. For example, since health and sustainability represent universal goals, these introduce natural unifying visions that provide meaning and purpose to people around the world. Since these visions apply to everyone, they may have the potential to motivate people to act collectively for the whole.

A vision for healthy sustainable living can evolve us internally beyond our everyday, special interest concerns. Instead of acting solely for our self in the context of our mortal existence, we can now act on behalf of our immortal existence. We intentionally contribute to others, the planet, and evolution. Our consciousness and actions attempt to improve our relationships in the world and sometimes live on in others who can evolve our consciousness and actions further. In this way, we can continue to evolve through others and evolutionary processes via our immortal existence. The energy, information, and matter that we change in our mortal life continue to evolve in the immortal nature of ongoing evolution.

Healthy Sustainable Living Models as Conscious Evolution Tools

Healthy Living Model

The healthy living model (see figure 5) facilitates individuals to perform, synergize, and balance their functioning across the twelve universal health dimensions. This model provides the necessary initial step to improve health and sustainability on the individual level (see Figure 18). Yet our personal health depends upon our individual functioning as well as on healthy functioning throughout the different levels of society, including the family, business, community, nation, and world levels. Therefore, we need all levels of society to operate in healthy sustainable manners for us to optimize our individual functioning.

Societal Healthy Living Model

The societal healthy living model (see figure 10) provides the tool necessary to expand healthy living to all levels of society. It enables us to comprehend how different levels of society operate with the health dimensions, as well as how the different levels affect each other (see Figure 18). For instance, if the family level has nearly half of marriages ending in divorce, then individual health, business performance, and community, national, and global functioning will all experience somewhat diminished health and sustainability due to the unhealthy dynamics associated with the devolution of the relationship.

Fortunately, the societal model serves to expand our consciousness into the worldcentric perspective. When we appreciate that healthy living occurs across the individual to the global levels, this challenges us to expand our consciousness. Although this worldcentric consciousness may be limited to our time that we spend working with the model, it promotes perceptions, decision making, and actions at progressively more sustainable levels.

Comprehensive Healthy Living Model

The comprehensive healthy living model (see figure 11) provides the means to assess and then intervene to improve healthy sustainable living on the worldcentric level. It introduces the opportunity for treatment interventions to help heal destruction already occurring (see Figure 18). It encourages prevention interventions to avoid potential destruction and supports the maintenance of our present functioning. Finally, wellness interventions promote our continued growth, and ultimately, our optimal performance. In these ways, we can consciously intervene and respect the natural growth, maintenance, and destruction processes inherent in evolution. We can then consciously work to maximize our health and sustainability, as we live within these larger evolutionary processes.

Evolutionary Ethical Living Model

While all the previous models are necessary and important, the evolutionary ethical living model is the most vital one for creating sustainable living. It provides a kosmocentric perspective that invites people to consider their lives in the context of all humanity, the planet, evolution, and *reality* as a whole. It enables us to transcend temporarily from any of the less inclusive stages of consciousness. We can then perceive *reality* from an evolutionary perspective that facilitates our ability to detect potential harm or destruction to our culture, species, and the biological and physical environments. Since our lives stand upon all these levels exhibited in this model, we must take responsibility for all these underlying levels, if we intend to stay on top of the world. If we choose not to embrace our evolutionary responsibilities, then our time on top of the world appears within five minutes of striking midnight according to the Doomsday Clock.

If our personal consciousness and actions provoke significant destruction to any of these levels of *reality*, then our lives can face real threats of devolution. As a consequence, we need to assess any potential harm to these foundational levels to our lives. We then need to avoid, prevent, or treat actions that threaten destruction on each of these evolutionary levels. Otherwise, we risk our own destruction.

Since the ethical living model portrays spiritual evolution as the ground from which all evolution arises, our responsibilities extend beyond our evolutionary work into reverence for the ground of being. In evolution we operate as cocreative, miniature gods at the cutting edge of creation. We produce more change in the world now than traditional random mutations. Therefore, we exist as spiritual human beings who inherently have responsibilities to all *reality*, or to God or Spirit as the source and the creation of *reality*. Consequently, we must evolve our consciousness beyond our self- and group-centered interests. We need to embrace our greatest responsibilities resonant with our highest spiritual and human potentials, so we cocreate for the benefit of the oneness of all.

An Integrated Model to Create a Healthy Sustainable Future via Conscious Evolution

In this section, I will describe a seven-step process of conscious evolution designed to create healthy sustainable living (see Figure 19). This integrated, healthy sustainable living model incorporates the four previous models into a comprehensive process to accelerate safe and effective, conscious evolution.

Before utilizing the models though, we need to unite consciously with the "Evolutionary Impulse" (Hamilton, 2012b). In this way we consciously activate our evolutionary self, so we can cocreate with *reality* from this universal perspective. Meanwhile, we can also activate our highest, most inclusive "Stages of Consciousness" to maximize the freedom and inclusiveness of our conscious evolution efforts. Since worldcentric and especially kosmocentric consciousness perceives *reality* fully enough for us to promote sustainability, we need to function at these levels. Fortunately, the models have been intentionally designed to provide worldcentric and kosmocentric perspectives.

The "Processes of Evolution" influence whether the actions chosen from the models will successfully generate positive change. For instance, if our creative action fails to move from the competitive arena of natural selection into the cooperative field in which we organize and order our creation, it will probably not lead to healthy sustainable functioning.

We improve our "Conscious Evolution" efforts when we intentionally shift beyond accidental and random outcomes and, instead, set specific goals to achieve. We can shift into transformational change territory when we follow visions intended for the whole of humanity and the world. In this case, the models and the vision coordinate to help create a successful future of healthy sustainable living.

Figure 19:
Integrated, Healthy Sustainable Living Model to Guide
Conscious Evolution into a Viable Future

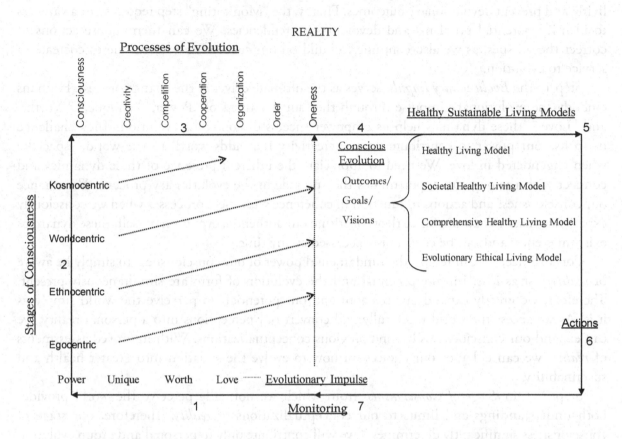

The "Healthy Sustainable Living Models" transport us into worldcentric or kosmocentric perspectives to evaluate the issues of our concern. We can assess, plan, and prioritize regarding how to transform the situation into improved health and sustainability. The "Actions" we then choose naturally emerge from the previous five steps. These actions support healthy sustainable living and prevent devolutionary outcomes. Finally, the "Monitoring" step requires our awareness to identify potential problems and devolutionary tendencies. We can then choose actions to correct these issues, as we also continue to build on our successes and continue to cocreate in service to evolution.

Step 1. The *Evolutionary Impulse* serves as the ultimate driver of the change process. Humans embody the evolutionary impulse through the four dynamics of "Power," "Unique," "Worth," and "Love." These dynamics help us empower successful conscious evolution. They challenge us to use our power to contribute unique creativity that adds worth to the world, especially when engendered in love. We need to appreciate the inherent presence of these dynamics and connect with the ongoing opportunities they provide in the evolutionary process. We enhance our consciousness and actions to function in coherence with these processes when we consciously experience these dynamics. Since they constitute our authentic, evolutionary self, these dynamics exist inherently and can be consciously accessed at any time.

For instance, we can realize the fundamental power of our consciousness to simply be aware of *reality* just as it is. Infinite potential and the evolution of form are simultaneously present. Therefore, we greatly expand our freedom and our potentials to perceive the world simply as it is. As we access the world more fully and convert our perceptions into a personal reality, we can expand our consciousness beyond previous conceptualizations. With improved assessments of *reality*, we can enhance our choices on how to evolve the situation into greater health and sustainability.

Step 2. Our *Stage of Consciousness* from which we normally perceive the world provides both understandings and limits to our conceptualizations of *reality*. Therefore, our stage of consciousness significantly determines if we will contribute only to personal and group evolution or also contribute consciously to the evolution of the world and all *reality*. For example, if we use egocentric or ethnocentric perspectives as our primary lenses, we may successfully cocreate for the benefit of our self or our group, as we unknowingly inflict harm on others and the environment that exist beyond our present interests. Consequently, we need to develop a worldcentric perspective in which we act to benefit others and the world, while we also protect them from harm. Ideally, we need to develop a kosmocentric perspective to maximize our perceptions of *reality* that, in turn, minimize our potentials to generate devolutionary processes that undermine our future.

Step 3. Conscious evolution can effectively follow the natural *Processes of Evolution*. Thus, we use our consciousness to stimulate creativity that competes in the selection processes to gain support and cooperation from others. We can then organize the multiple relationships involved to generate a new interdependent order that culminates in functioning as a more unified whole. This process converts our separate consciousness or actions through the use of relationships with others and the world to generate a more complex oneness of functioning. When perceived consistent with a worldcentric or, ideally, a kosmocentric perspective, the creative process increasingly contributes to healthy sustainable living.

Step 4. Evolution can proceed randomly and accidentally or we can progress systematically through *Conscious Evolution*. Traditionally, conscious evolution has occurred largely through the attainment of goals (usually short-term, special interest planning goals). Nevertheless, I propose that we now need to shift into visionary planning to overcome the devolutionary side effects often associated with traditional, special interest goal-setting. Henceforth we need visions to evolve the separate parts, the relationships, and the whole functioning of humanity and the planet. The proposed vision for healthy sustainable living meets this inclusive criterion. In addition, it builds upon the natural motivations within people to enjoy health rather than suffer sickness as well as sustain life rather than devolve into death. Consequently, the universal motivations toward health and sustainability combine to produce a natural vision to guide and motivate us into the future. We can then use short-term goals to supplement our long-term vision. Conscious evolution needs visionary goals that integrate the separate special interests and their interdependent relationships in order to create health and sustainability for all.

Step 5. The *Healthy Sustainable Living Models* promote successful conscious evolution. Health and sustainability function at the core, as necessary processes in human evolution. Therefore, they introduce a universal value system to guide our conscious evolution. Humans and evolution must function in interdependent relationships that promote mutual health and sustainability. The four models serve like maps to guide our attempts for growth and maintenance. In addition, the models help identify potential harm and devolutionary outcomes, so we can choose further actions that contribute to evolution.

Each of these models provides an important visualization of health that expands upon the previous model. For instance, individual healthy living relies on the societal healthy living model to assess healthy functioning across all twelve dimensions and across all levels of society. In this way, we can consciously choose how to grow, maintain, and heal health for individuals and groups across all levels of society. We possess a comprehensive methodology to assess and systematically confront any human problem. The evolutionary ethical living model provides the most comprehensive perspective as it includes all levels of humanity, of evolution, and the potential of all. Therefore, this final model provides a kosmocentric perspective on how to assess the benefits and harm associated with any action across *reality*. As a result, this ethical model provides an all-encompassing map that highlights how to create health and sustainability.

We expand our potency with the models when we connect with the ever-present dynamics of the evolutionary impulse and then intentionally access our highest stage of consciousness. The "models invite us to experience temporary states of consciousness that are similar to or in harmony with worldcentric and kosmocentric levels" (Morelli, 2012). The more consistently that we enter into these states, the more likely we will eventually learn to act at these levels of awareness in our everyday lives without the assistance of the models. We also enhance our success with the models when we create and follow the natural processes of evolution. For instance, we can share our separate creation within cooperative relationships in attempts to foster more organized, orderly functioning that contributes to the ultimate vision for healthy sustainable living.

Step 6. From our assessment in step 5, we can choose *Actions* that we can initiate with greater confidence of their evolutionary potentials. We can prioritize and coordinate the actions across the health dimensions and across all levels of *reality*. These actions need to support the growth and maintenance of ourselves and humanity, while preventing any significant devolutionary harm. Recall that we stand on the top of all the human and planetary evolution systems. Therefore, we must prevent harm in these underlying foundations to our lives if we expect to remain standing.

Consequently, we have to expand from our traditional personal and cultural growth preferences and prioritize the prevention of devolutionary harm as our most important mission.

Metaphorically, we have to act like evolutionary parents who prioritize safety first so growth can then freely follow. Conversely, we have to shift from the child role in which self-interest growth and immediate gratification frequently dominate. The capitalist economy depends on and currently rewards such special interest growth over growth that responsibly develops the collective and the whole. Therefore, we need to evolve personally and institutionally to initiate actions that foster health and sustainability as more important than, but inclusive of special interest gains and economic profits.

Step 7. *Monitoring* the consequences of our actions for evolutionary and devolutionary outcomes enable conscious evolution to proceed. In a sense, monitoring in step 7 operates like a miniature evolutionary process that occurs within the larger evolutionary scene. In this case our consciousness observes evolution in motion and converts the observation into our limited personal reality that we comprehend as the "truth" of the situation. Our unique version of *reality* then introduces mutations via our consciousness and our actions into the world. Thus, our limited personal reality evolves internally and serves to mutate the larger evolutionary processes.

When we increase the inclusiveness of our consciousness, we more accurately and fully embrace *reality* as it is. Our cocreative powers increase. Through the use of our miniature god capabilities we can also introduce intentions, such as to create a better world. Ideally, this intention to contribute to a better world applies to us, our groups, all humanity, as well as to all life forms, the planet, evolution, and to *reality* itself. We can then choose actions to cocreate based on our vision of the future, in this case, our vision for creating healthy sustainable living.

Whenever we detect successes and failures associated with our cocreation efforts, we can adeptly introduce information and action modifications to build on the successes and stop, prevent, or avoid any devolutionary actions. If a destructive result starts to appear or seems likely on any of the foundational levels of physical, biological, and human evolution, then we need to stop the actions. In such cases, the long-term consequences on these deeper levels take priority over benefits accrued on higher levels of cultural, societal, and personal functioning. This priority shift away from traditional planning approaches occurs because lower level devolution means that all higher levels will likely also suffer devolution. Accordingly, serious damage to any underlying level that supports our miniature god perch on top of the evolutionary pyramid threatens damages and potential devolution to us.

Monitoring represents the ongoing process of conscious observation, so our personal evolution and the evolution of the whole have the opportunity to unite in greater oneness. In other words, monitoring provides additional information to increase the accuracy of our perceptions of *reality*. We can then more easily transcend our normal perceptions of separateness and engage in the relationships that unite us with the whole. A natural goal emerges in this process in which we strive for greater oneness with *reality* as we perceive and act in increasing harmony with all that exists. As a result, our mission for conscious evolution becomes clear in that we work to create healthy sustainable living with all that exists and has the potential to exist, so we can continue as cocreators on this great evolutionary journey.

References

Ardagh, Arjuna. *The Translucent Revolution: How People Just Like You Are Waking Up and Changing the World*. Novato, CA: New World Library, 2005.

Bougsty, Tom. *Healthy Living: How to Create a Personal Health Plan*. E-book available on Tom Bougsty's web site at Healthy-Sustainable-Living.com, 2012.

Bougsty-Marshall, Skye. Personal communications. November 5, 2012.

Brown, Daniel P. *Pointing Out the Great Way The Stages of Meditation in the Mahamudra Tradition*. Somerville, MA: Wisdom Publications, Inc., 2006.

Bureau of Labor Statistics. www.bls.gov/news.release/empsit.nr0.htm. 2011.

Bureau of Labor Statistics. http://www.bls.gov/news.release/empsit.t15.htm, 2012.

Campbell, Colin J. "About Peak Oil/Understanding Peak Oil." www.peakoil.net/about-peak-oil, accessed April 18, 2009.

Centers for Disease Control and Prevention Office on Smoking and Health (CDC OSH). "Best Practices for Comprehensive Tobacco Control Programs," August 1999. Atlanta GA: National Center for Chronic Disease Prevention and Health Promotion, Office on Smoking and Health, 1999.

Centers for Disease Control and Prevention's Office on Smoking and Health (CDC OSH). "Investing in Tobacco Control: A Guide for State Decision-makers," presented in a satellite conference, February 15, 2001.

Centers for Disease Control and Prevention. "Best Practices for Comprehensive Tobacco Control Programs," 2007. Atlanta: US Department of Health and Human Services, Centers for Disease Control and Prevention, National Center for Chronic Disease Prevention and Health Promotion, Office on Smoking and Health, October, 2007a.

Centers for Disease Control and Prevention. Rising Health Care Costs Are Unsustainable. www.cdc.gov/workplacehealthpromotion/businesscase/reasons/rising.html, 2007b, accessed September 11, 2012.

Centers for Disease Control and Prevention. Obesity and Overweight. www.cdc.gov/nchs/fastats/overwt.htm, 2007–08, accessed September 7, 2012.

Centers for Disease Control and Prevention. Marriage and Divorce. www.cdc.gov/nchs/fastats/divorce.htm, 2009a, accessed September 7, 2012.

Centers for Disease Control and Prevention. "The Power of Prevention Chronic Disease … the Public Health Challenge of the Twenty-First Century." www.cdc.gov/chronicdisease/pdf/2009-Power-of-Prevention.pdf, 2009b, accessed September 14, 2012.

Centers for Disease Control and Prevention. "Chronic Disease Prevention and Health Promotion." www.cdc.govchronicdisease/overview/index.htm, accessed September 14, 2012.

Centers for Medicare and Medicaid Services. National Health Expenditure Fact Sheet. www.cms.gov/Research-Statistics-Data-and-Systems/Statistics-Trends-and-Reports/NationalHealthExpendData/NHE-Fact-Sheet.html, 2009, accessed September 11, 2012.

Childre, Doc Lew, Howard Martin, and Donna Beech. *The HeartMath Solution: The Institute of HeartMath's Revolutionary Program for Engaging the Power of the Heart's Intelligence.* New York: HarperOne, 2000.

Chopra, Deepak. *The Spontaneous Fulfillment of Desire, Harnessing the Infinite Power of Coincidence.* New York: Harmony Books, 2003.

Cohen, Andrew. *Evolutionary Enlightenment A New Path to Spiritual Awakening.* New York: SelectBooks, Inc., 2012.

Cohen, Andrew and Ken Wilber. "The Guru and the Pandit: Following the Grain of the Kosmos: States, Stages, Selves, and Directionality of Development. "What Is Enlightenment?" Lenox, MA: Moksha Press, Issue 25, May–July 2004, 44–53.

Commonweal. What is the Precautionary Principle? http://www.commonweal.org/programs/precautionary-principle.html, September 14, 2012.

Daly, John, Chris Martenson, Keith Fitz-Gerald, and Kent Moors. "The Pyramid Crisis: Protect Yourself from the Greatest Threat to Your Financial Security and Way of Life." http://moneymappress.com/pro/Pyramid0712MMR.php?code=LPYRN801&n=PYRAMIDMMR49EADMMP, accessed August 2, 2012.

Department of the Air Force. Final Environmental Planning Technical Report Public Services and Facilities. Peacekeeper missile deployment, January 1984.

Dowd, Michael. *Thank GOD for Evolution: How the Marriage of Science and Religion Will Transform Your Life and Our World.* San Francisco, CA: Council Oak Books, 2007.

Edmonson, Donald. "Had a Heart Attack? Watch Out for PTSD." *Daily Health News,* Bottom Line Publications, September 11, 2012.

Elgin, Duane. *Voluntary Simplicity toward a Way of Life that Is Outwardly Simple, Inwardly Rich*. New York: Harper, Second Edition, 2010.

Fenner, Peter. *Radiant Mind, Awakening Unconditioned Awareness*. Boulder, C0: Sounds True, Inc., 2007.

Global Issues. Poverty Facts and Stats. http://www.globalissues.org/article/26/poverty-facts-and-stats, Anup Shah, September 20, 2010.

Global Oneness Summit. http://www.globalonenesssummit.com. Agents of Conscious Evolution Training. The Shift Network, Barbara Marx Hubbard and Stephen Dinan, 2011.

Hamilton, Craig. "Integral Enlightenment: Awakening to an Evolutionary Relationship to Life." Integral Enlightenment training, events@integralenlightenment.com, 2010.

Hamilton, Craig. Meditation for Evolutionaries Gathering. Integral Enlightenment training, 369-B Third Street, Suite 302, San Rafael, CA. 94901, July 29, 2012a.

Hamilton, Craig. "Academy for Evolutionaries." Awakening the Evolutionary Self, http://integralenlightenment.com/, September 15, 2012b.

Hanson, Rick. "Buddha's Brain: The Practical Neuroscience of Happiness, Love and Wisdom." CMI Education Institute, http://www.pesi.com/, Interactive webcast, January 28, 2012.

Hartmann, Thom. *Unequal Protection The Rise of Corporate Dominance and the Theft of Human Rights*. www.rodalestore.com, 2004.

Healthy People 2020. Tobacco Use. www.healthypeople.gov/2020/topicsobjectives2020/overview.aspx?topicid=41, accessed September 14, 2012.

Helliwell, John F., Layard, Richard, and Sachs, Jeff, Eds. World Happiness Report. Commissioned for the United Nations Conference on Happiness on April 2, 2012 (mandated by the General Assembly of the United Nations), The Earth Institute, Columbia University, New York, 2012.

http://www.lifeaftertheoilcrash.net/. April 10, 2009.

Hubbard, Barbara Marx. *Conscious Evolution: Awakening the Power of Our Social Potential*. Novato, CA: New World Library, 1998.

Hubbard, Barbara Marx. *Emergence: The Shift from Ego to Essence*. Charlottesville, VA: Hampton Roads Publishing Company, Inc., 2001.

Hubbard, Barbara Marx. "Agent of Conscious Evolution Training." http://birth2012.com/sites/birth2012.com/files/Birth2012Activation.pdf, accessed March 22, 2011.

Hubbard, Barbara Marx. *Birth 2012 and beyond: Humanity's Great Shift to the Age of Conscious Evolution*. www.shiftmovement.com, Shift Books, 2012.

Human Development Reports. Human Development Report 2011 Sustainability and Equity: A Better Future for All. hdr.undp.org/en/reports/global/hdr1998/chapters/, accessed September 15, 2012.

Institute of Medicine. "State Programs Can Reduce Tobacco Use. A Report of the National Cancer Policy Board." Washington, DC: National Research Council, 2000.

Jones, Lola. *Things Are Going Great In My Absence: How to Let Go and Let the Divine Do the Heavy Lifting.* www.divineopenings.com, 2006.

Leeb, Stephen. http://www.completeinvestor.com/. April 21, 2009.

Liptak, Adam. "US prison population dwarfs that of other nations." The *New York Times*, April 23, 2008.

MacLean, Paul. *The Triune Brain in Evolution, Role in Paleocerebral Functions.* New York: Plenum Press, 1990.

McIntosh, Steve. *Integral Consciousness and the Future of Evolution How the Integral Worldview Is Transforming Politics, Culture and Spirituality.* St. Paul, MN: Paragon House, 2007.

McIntosh, Steve. "Evolution's Purpose: The Ever-Widening Realization of Beauty, Truth, and Goodness." Interview with Terry Patten, http://beyondawakeningseries@e.evolvingwisdom.com, August 26, 2012.

McTaggart, Lynne. *The FIELD the Quest for the Secret Force of the Universe.* New York: HarperCollins Publishers, 2002.

McTaggart, Lynne. *The BOND Connecting through the Space between Us.* New York: Free Press, Simon & Schuster, Inc., 2011.

Milken Institute. "An Unhealthy America: The Economic Impact of Chronic Disease." http://www.chronicdiseaseimpact.com/ebcd.taf?cat=disease&type=heart, 2003a, accessed September 7, 2012.

Milken Institute. "An Unhealthy America: The Economic Impact of Chronic Disease." http://www.chronicdiseaseimpact.com/ebcd.taf?cat=disease&type=emotional, 2003b, accessed September 7, 2012.

Milken Institute. "An Unhealthy America: The Economic Impact of Chronic Disease." http://www.chronicdiseaseimpact.com/ebcd.taf?cat=method, 2003c, accessed September 9, 2012.

Morelli, Marco. Personal communication. August 21, 2012.

Muller, Richard. "Koch Brother-Funded Climate Change Denier Changes His Tune." Thom Hartmann Program, Free Speech TV, July 31, 2012.

My Budget 360. Top 1 percent Control 42 percent of Financial Wealth in the U.S. http://www.mybudget360.com, 2011.

National Center for Chronic Disease Prevention and Control. The Power of Prevention Chronic Disease … the Public Health Challenge of the Twenty-First Century. http://www.cdc.gov/chronicdisease/pdf/2009-Power-of-Prevention.pdf, 2009, accessed September 11, 2012.

NRDC. Fuel Facts: "Governments Should Phase Out Fossil Fuel Subsidies or Risk Lower Economic Growth, Delayed Investment in Clean Energy and Unnecessary Climate Change Pollution." http://www.nrdc.org/energy/files/fossilfuel4.pdf. July 4, 2012.

O'Day, Candice. "Open-Ended Knowledge Creation." Interview with Terry Patten, http://beyondawakeningseries@e.evolvingwisdom.com, April 29, 2012.

Ortner, Nick. Tapping Summit. http://www.thetappingsolution.com/2012tappingworldsummit/2012_upgrade.html, 2012.

Pappas, Stephanie and LiveScience. "Doomsday Clock Moved One Minute Closer to Midnight." *Scientific American*, January 10, 2012.

Patten, Terry. "A New Spiritual Horizon." Interview with Craig Hamilton, http://beyondawakeningseries@e.evolvingwisdom.com, June 3, 2012.

Peak Oil. Info and Strategies. http://www.oildecline.com/, April 18, 2009.

Phipps, Carter. *Evolutionaries Unlocking the Spiritual and Cultural Potential of Science's Greatest Idea*. NY: Harper-Perennial, 2012.

Polya, Gideon. http://www.green-blog.org/2008/06/14/pollutants-from-coal-based-electricity-generation-kill-170000-people-annually/. Accessed April 14, 2012.

Stern, N. "Stern Review: The Economics of Climate Change." http://www.hm-treasury.gov.uk/stern_review_report.htm, 2006.

Swimme, Brian. Interview with Craig Hamilton. Evolutionary Life Transformation Program, December 7, 2010.

Swimme, Brian and Mary Evelyn Tucker. *Journey of the Universe*. New Haven, CT: Yale University Press, 2011.

TEEB. "The Economics of Ecosystems and Biodiversity for National and International Policy Makers—Summary: Responding to the Value of Nature 2009." http://www.teebtest.org/teeb-study-and-reports/overview-of-teeb-studies/2009, accessed October 29, 2012.

The International Union for Conservation of Nature (IUCN). "Red List Species Extinction: The Facts." http://cmsdata.iucn.org/downloads/species_extinction_05_2007.pdf, accessed September 14, 2012.

The World Bank. "Rio+20: natural capital accounting and the wealth of countries." June 15, 2012a, http://www.worldbank.org/en/news/2012/05/30/rio-20-natural-capital-accounting-feature, accessed September 14, 2012.

The World Bank. "Sustainable Development: Natural Capital Accounting." June 22, 2012b, http://web.worldbank.org/Wbsite/External/Topics/Extsdnet/0,,contentMDK:23168586~pagePK:64885161~piPK:64884432~theSitePK:5929282,00.html, accessed September 14, 2012.

US Census Bureau. "Income, Poverty, and Health Insurance in the United States: 2010—Highlights." http://www.census.gov/hhes/www/poverty/data/incpovhlth/2010/highlights.html, accessed August 21, 2012.

US Department of Health and Human Services. Agency for Healthcare Research and Quality. http://www.ahrq.gov/research/ria19/expendra.htm, September 14, 2012.

US Energy & Information Administration (EIA). Energy in Brief. "What Everyone Should Know about Energy." http://www.eia.gov/energy_in_brief/foreign_oil_dependence.cfm, September 1, 2010.

US Energy & Information Administration (EIA). "Energy in Brief. What Everyone Should Know about Energy." http://www.eia.gov/energy_in_brief/foreign_oil_dependence.cfm, May 6, 2011.

US Environmental Protection Agency. http://www.epa.gov/crossstaterule/ Cross-State Air Pollution Rule (CSAPR). April 7, 1012.

Wilber, Ken. "Kosmic Consciousness," Boulder, CO: Sounds True, 2003.

Wilber, Ken. *The Simple Feeling of Being: Embracing Your True Nature.* Compiled and edited by Mark Palmer, Sean Hargens, Vipassana Esbjörn, and Adam Leonard, Boston, MA: Shambhala, 2004.

Wilber, Ken. *Integral Spirituality: A Startling New Role for Religion in the Modern and Postmodern World.* Boston, MA: Integral Books, 2006.

Wilber, Ken. "Creating an Integral Culture." *Beyond Awakening,* Terry Patten, http://beyondawakeningseries.com/blog/archive/, September 16, 2010.

Wilson, Robert Anton. "Information is doubling faster all the time." http://realneo.us/content/information-doubling-faster-all-time, Quest-News-Service, May 20, 2009.

Yarra Valley Climate Action Group. "Pollution Deaths from Fossil Fuel-based Power Plants." http://sites.google.com/site/yarravalleyclimateactiongroup/pollution-deaths-from-fossil-fuel-based-power-plants, April 14, 2012.